PSYCHOTHERAPY
OF THE
RELIGIOUS PATIENT

PSYCHOTHERAPY OF THE RELIGIOUS PATIENT

Edited by

MOSHE HALEVI SPERO, Ph.D.

Assistant Professor and Chairman (on leave)
Department of Individual and Social Behavior
Notre Dame College of Ohio
Senior Lecturer, School of Social Work
Bar Ilan University
Ramat Gan, Israel
Co-editor, **Journal of Psychology and Judaism**

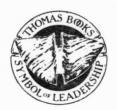

CHARLES C THOMAS • PUBLISHER
Springfield • Illinois • U.S.A.

Published and Distributed Throughout the World by

CHARLES C THOMAS • PUBLISHER

2600 South First Street

Springfield, Illinois 62717

With THOMAS BOOKS *careful attention is given to all details of manufacturing and
design. It is the Publisher's desire to present books that are satisfactory as to their physical
qualities and artistic possibilities and appropriate for their particular use.* THOMAS
BOOKS *will be true to those laws of quality that assure a good name and good will.*

Printed in the United States of America
Q-R-3

Library of Congress Cataloging in Publication Data

Main entry under title:
Psychotherapy of the religious patient.

   Bibliography: p.
   1. Psychotherapy — Religious   aspects.
2. Psychotherapy   patients — Religious   life.   I. Spero,
Moshe HaLevi.
RC 455.4.R4P79   1984   616.89'14   84-8810
ISBN 0-398-05058-9

Dedicated to Yehudit
and to three good friends,
Aryeh, Chaim Tzvi, and Zanvel

CONTRIBUTORS

Seymour W. Applebaum, M.D.
Adjunct Professor of Psychiatry & Psychopathology, Wurzweiler School of Social Work, Yeshiva University, New York
Private Practice
118-80 Metropolitan Ave.
Kew Gardens, NY 11415

Paul R. Bindler, Ph.D.
Clinical Instructor in Psychiatry, Mt. Sinai School of Medicine, C.U.N.Y.
Director, Biofeedback and Strees Management Center, National Institute of the Psychotherapies, New York
Editor, *Intercom*
Clinical Psychologist, Private Practice
1060 East 26th St.
Brooklyn, NY 11210

David Terry Bradford, M.Th., Ph.D.
Postdoctoral Fellow in Neuropsychology, Oregon State Hospital
3626 Myrla Court St.
Salem, OR 97302

David A. Halperin, M.D.
Assistant Clinical Professor in Psychiatry, Mt. Sinai School of Medicine, C.U.N.Y.
Staff, Cult Hotline and Treatment Program, Jewish Board of Family and Children's Services, New York
Private Practice
20 West 86th Street
New York, NY 10024

Paul Kahn, Ph.D.
Rabbi, Young Israel of Mapelton Park, Brooklyn
Editor, *Proceedings of the Associations of Orthodox Jewish Scientists*
Supervisor, School Psychologists, New York Board of Education
Clinical Psychologist, Private Practice
1460 West 9th St.
Brooklyn, NY 11204

Robert J. Lovinger, Ph.D.

Faculty, Central Michigan University

Clinical Psychologist, Private Practice

714 South Main St.
Mt. Pleasant, MI 48858

John R. Peteet, M.D.

Associate in Medicine (Psychiatry), Brigham & Women's Hospital, Boston

Instructor in Psychiatry, Harvard Medical School

75 Francis St.
Boston, MA 02115

Leon Salzman, M.D.

Clinical Professor of Psychiatry, Georgetown University Medical School

Private Practice

1800 R St. NW
Washington, DC 20009

Ira F. Scharff, M.S.W., A.C.S.W.

Supervisor, Westchester Jewish Community Services

Adjunct Associate Professor, New York University School of Social Work

Faculty, Institute for Contemporary Psychotherapy

9 Hidden Glen Lane
Monsey, NY 10952

Moshe Halevi Spero, Ph.D.

Assistant Professor and Chairman (on leave), Department of Individual and Social Behavior, Notre Dame College of Ohio

Senior Lecturer, School of Social Work, Bar Ilan University, Israel

Co-Editor, *Journal of Psychology and Judaism*

Child & Adolescent Therapist, Private Practice

3808 Severn Rd.
Cleveland, OH 44118

PREFACE

THIS text has been compiled for the mental health practitioner who is interested in the psychotherapeutic treatment of religious patients. While some general texts are available which discuss the philosophical relationship between psychotherapy and religious beliefs, and some others which focus upon developmental aspects of healthy and pathological religiosity, the present text is devoted to the diagnosis and treatment of psychologically disturbed or conflict-ridden religious personalities.

The authors of these chapters have strived dilligently not only to present portraits of their patients' troubled psychosocial and religious lives, but also the specific techniques they have utilized in the effort to effect positive change in their patients. The reader may not agree with every approach. Some techniques are more directive than select readers might be accustomed to; others are applied to clinical populations from which generalizations may be unwarranted. Finally, the authors reflect different degrees and levels of experience with treating religious patients. Nonetheless, the wealth of clinical material and insight gathered here should provide a fruitful data base for comparisons, reflections, and further hypothesizing.

I am grateful to the numerous authors who participated in this venture, who accepted favorably my editorial suggestions and pre-rogatives, and who paused to think critically about the work they do with this unique set of patients and to share their observations with others. I am indebted to Mr. Payne Thomas for publishing these papers and for fulfilling my expectations of excellence in the final product.

I am most thankful for the support of Notre Dame College of

Ohio, its president, Sr. Mary Martha Reinhard, S.N.D., and academic dean, Sr. Mary Donald Ann Dunham, S.N.D., who encouraged me to teach the concepts I derived from my clinical experience and who deeply appreciated my particular area of interest in psychology and religion. Thanks also are due to Mrs. Marie Kuret who patiently typed and retyped this manuscript. Finally, in that unique category, I express continued love and affection to my dear wife and children who provide support of the most important kind and quality.

CONTENTS

Section Three — TRANSFERENCE, COUNTERTRANSFERENCE, AND THE ALLIANCE

Section Four—CASE STUDIES IN PSYCHOTHERAPY

PSYCHOTHERAPY
OF THE
RELIGIOUS PATIENT

Section One
INTRODUCTION

Chapter 1

SELECTED METACLINICAL PROBLEMS IN THE PSYCHOTHERAPEUTIC TREATMENT OF THE DISORDERED RELIGIOUS PERSONALITY

MOSHE HALEVI SPERO, Ph.D.

T HE papers presented in this text address the practical intersect
between psychology, psychiatry, and religion — a relationship
which has enjoyed intensive examination from theoretical and philosophical viewpoints (Pattison, 1978a, b). In 1937, Robert Knight
claimed that the psychoanalytic treatment of a religious minister was
a noteworthy event. In 1964, Mann reported his colleagues' obser-
vation that the practicing psychoanalyst rarely encounters the deeply
and authentically committed religious patient. Yet, since that time,
psychotherapists and lay and religious counselors have sporadically
reported the diagnosis and treatment of patients whose religious beliefs and practices are deeply enmeshed in their core psychological
and interpersonal conflicts.

CASE STUDY APPROACH

The literature up to and including the present has never contained an abundance of clinical material presenting in sufficient detail the specific diagnostic and treatment procedures used with

religious patients. The vast majority of papers dealing with the topic are theoretical or offer by way of clinical illustration radically abbreviated vignettes of limited practical utility. All too often, these papers are written with the belief that if the reader can appreciate the clinical summary and the brief theoretical discussion he will automatically be able to conduct successful psychotherapy with similar kinds of patients. In fact, as Spence has lamented recently, this frequently is not the case. First, the subgroup of religious patients includes a variety of types and qualities of religiosity as well as types of psychopathology for which specific technique cannot always be generalized from the few existing papers. Second, the nuances of technique usually are not amply conveyed let alone are learned from telescoped case vignettes, and our experience alone tells us that there is much that transpires when working with such patients which challenges our *prima facie* clinical attitudes and technical approaches. It is thus necessary to develop a more detailed case approach for transmitting the skills acquired in working with the religious patient.

Aside from other kinds of research on the religious personality, the clinical or case study method provides a particularly "solid basis for understanding the place of religion in the dynamics of human life" (Casey, 1938, p. 452). This is so for at least four reasons, gleaned from the work of Rizzuto (1974, 1979) and others: (1) the clinical approach allows the psychotherapist to use the patient's vocabulary to understand the historical roots of the patient's belief or lack of belief; (2) it deals with the patient as a concrete historical being in the here and now rather than as an abstract, and deals with the patient's experiences as they occur; (3) it permits the use of interpretations applied to the internal consistency of the patient's life history, object relationships, relation to God, within the context of the past and the present; and (4) it permits one to understand the private God (or "God representation") of each person.

The religious patient presents the clinician with certain unique technical and ethical dilemmas. If it is the case in general that therapists' values influence their patients directly and indirectly (Bergin, 1980; Ehrlich & Wiener, 1961; Krasner, 1982; London, 1964; Pattison, 1968; Wile, 1977; Wolberg, 1977), requiring conscious efforts to understand, predict, and modulate these influences, this is certainly the case with the highly guarded and bias-ridden domain of religious values and beliefs about religious values.

Additional factors make many therapists and mental health workers hesitant to cooperate with religious clientele, or motivate uncautious enthusiasm for treating such persons, manifest in a reactive tendency to treat such persons as if their religiosity was irrelevant to the basic personality disorder. These factors include simple lack of knowledge about specific patients' religious systems, lack of familiarity with the psychology of the religious personality, countertransference reactions based in neurotic determinants in the therapist's personality, and conscious biases based on ethical and ideological precommitments.

DISTINGUISHING NEUROTIC VERSUS HEALTHY RELIGIOSITY

The analyses selected for this text seek clear distinctions between neurotogenic, destructive, or maladaptive religious belief and practice, on the one hand, and what by comparison are mature or authentic religious beliefs and practices even when the latter coexist with other forms of disturbance in the religious personality. Sometimes the distinction is obvious. Sometimes the distinction is drawn explicitly by the therapist and sometimes only implicitly. Some therapists share with the patient their assessment of the patient's religiosity while others do not. Nevertheless, it is crucial that the distinction be made since only disordered religiosity is the rightful target of psychotherapy or behavior modification, and yet *all* of the patient's religiosity may be a focal point at different stages of therapy.

This task is often complicated by the influence of a countervailing notion that the presence of infantile elements in religious belief *per se* is qualitatively and genetically identical with the dynamic infantile or neurotic elements in human personality. The impact of this notion is best illustrated by the once widely-held clinical view that evidence of religiosity in a personality suggests the existence of immature or infantile ego functioning. Yet it simply has not been proven that commitment to a religion with infantile components necessarily means that the believer is similarly fixated at or has failed to grow beyond an infantile level.

In fact, while infantile elements of personality can actively exert a regressive influence on autonomous ego functioning and overall behavior, appropriately neutralized or satisfied infantile elements can also be assimilated into healthy intrapsychic structures and autonomous functioning. It is thus to be expected that certain qualities of religious belief reflect failure to achieve completely healthy psychological development or the achievement of secondary autonomous qualities relative to neurotic personality structure. However, this does not rule out the ego's potential to also achieve some and perhaps many healthy benefits from these same qualities of religious belief. Most important, so-called unhealthy or dysautonomous religiosity generally reflects the disordered uses to which conflicted individuals put their religious beliefs and habits rather than a basic inadequacy in the religious belief system as such. At the same time, one cannot ignore the prevalence in contemporary times of certain religious cults that are so wholly and purposely oriented toward the conflicted and confused aspects of vulnerable persons as to deserve the label of "destructive" or "regressive" faith (Halperin, 1983; Pattison, 1980; Pruyser, 1977; Shapiro, 1977). And even in the case of such forms of religiosity, salubrious effects on personality have been reported (Galanter, *et al*, 1979; cf. Spero, 1982).

Stark's summary of studies on psychopathology and religious commitment is most cogent (1971): "Psychopathology seems to impede the manifestation of conventional religious beliefs and practices. Far from being especially apt to turn to faith in order to seek psychic comforts for their psychological afflictions, the neurotic and mentally ill seem to be significantly less likely to exhibit conventional religious commitment." When religious belief is adopted to disguise or even resolve deeper psychological disorder, the disguise is generally transparent or the resolution only apparent and mediocre. It is usually in such instances that the psychotherapist is called upon to trace the dysautonomous qualities of religiosity to their disordered determinants, to apply interventive methods to such factors, and, if possible, to enhance the individual's receptivity to more mature or conflict-free religious experiences.

The distinction between mature and immature religious beliefs depends upon accepting a set of assumptions common to contemporary psychology and religion on the general definition of interpersonal and individual mental well-being. This is primarily accomplished by highlighting the synthesis between certain basic psychological definitions of health and those espoused by most conventional religions. But this approach has two limitations. First, it recasts in psychiatric or psychological terms what essentially are religious or theological definitions of healthy mind and spirit. Such translation may deemphasize the specific historical, ethical, and valuational schemes within which a given religion incorporates its psychosocial norms. The problem of diagnosing homosexuality as a sexual perversion illustrates this problem. Psychiatry and the Judao-Christian ethic agree on many general definitions of mental health, yet whereas psychiatry views homosexuality as not necessarily aberrant, based on certain kinds of empirical evidence, Judaism and most Christian denominations view homosexuality as a moral and psychological disturbance regardless of empirical considerations.

For another example, Paul Meehl writes that the clinician examines the appropriateness and logic of the patient's religiosity the same way one looks at the appropriateness and logic of anything else the patient says or does. "What [the therapist] is doing, wittingly or not, is to tease out internal disharmonies within the patient's discourse. Whatever one's view may be regarding the ultimate source of moral concepts, it is obvious that logic and consistency within the moral system which the patient espouses is part of the patient's reality. I am saying that to commit a fallacy, or permit an inconsistency in one's thinking about values, is not fundamentally different from making a mistake in arithmetic or reacting irrationally on a transference basis"(1959, p. 258).

However, not all religious beliefs are logical the way arithmetic formuli are. While there may be no value in holding on to the the belief that $2+2=5$ and no real truth to the patient's perception that the therapist is "like" his father, there may be from the standpoint of the particular religion special qualities gained even from the disordered religious beliefs. For example, Judaism may accept that a religious homosexual's anxiety about discovery or his tormenting fantasies about paternal castration merit modification so that he can be free of these — but it would not accept to remove all of his anxiety and guilt about homosexuality, or his belief that he may be punished by God, inasmuch as Judaism considers homosexuality something to feel guilty about. How willing or able are clinicians to differentiate between these types of guilt or anxiety? Consider also the case of the obsessive-compulsive Christian Scientist reported by Cohen and Smith (1976), whose successful treatment cost her Christian Science beliefs. It is likely that Christian Science itself may have valued the patient's illness as an opportunity for the patient to test her religious faith. Even if the therapists who treated her acted appropriately from the standpoint of general definitions of mental health, did they act appropriately in *not* helping her to explore the possible religious meanings of her symptom from the standpoint of her religion?

A second problem is that clinicians tend to speak in terms of religion or religious process in general, with the assumption that distinctions drawn between mature and immature religiosity are sufficiently broad to include most established religious systems. This generates relatively loose criteria against which the clinician gauges "obviously" mature religiosity and "obviously" pathogenic religiosity. In fact, such criteria may not detect subtle forms of disorder which only emerge clearly against the context of full knowledge of the norms and rituals of a specific religion. Alternatively, such criteria may catch myriad idiosyncratic expressions of religious belief which are in fact *bona fide* rather than fantastical expressions of human need though they may have no comparible forms or source in any of the well-known conventional religious systems. If our response to this problem is that we must perforce utilize universal norms, then one has committed precisely the reduction clinicans so often are accused of by religion.

There is yet another problem inherent in clinical distinctions between mature and immature religiosity. Having accepted that only pathogenic religiosity is the rightful target of psychotherapy, it becomes additionally necessary to offer dynamic formulations of the development of normal, healthy religious belief, formulations which are related to but are not exhausted by psychosexual or psychosocial or object-relational descriptors. In other words, clinical intervention with the religious patient must proceed from a scheme which recognizes that there can be normal as well as pathological religious beliefs even in the psychologically disturbed individual, and which causes one to think about how certain basic psychological needs (the need for symbolism, for transitional spheres, etc.) are being met or expressed by persons who are not religious. Moreover, such formulations need to address the developmental processes during religious conversion as well as during the transition among different levels of religious commitment (Grock, 1962; Rizzuto, 1979, p. 358).

METACLINICAL DILEMMAS

Elsewhere, I stated regarding the religious patient (Spero, 1980, p. 203): "A therapist would be as ill-advised in failing to accept the patient as a religious individual as he would be in refusing to accept the patient as a speaking, thinking, and emoting being. If the patient perceives himself as religious, one aids the patient to experience religion in a healthier light. The therapeutic concern is how a patient functions as an individual with his or her given modes of expression." While this approach is compatible with that formulated by many of the workers whose essays appear in these pages, it requires amplification in a way that underscores some specific dilemmas therapists working with religious patients need to consider throughout the course of their work.

First, it seems the case as a general principle that disordered religiosity is an expression of disordered psychological need, whether or not the religious system itself is mature or otherwise. However, one must keep in mind that there are behaviors which are disordered only from the standpoint of the religion and not from the standpoint of contemporary psychiatric opinion (e.g., homosexuality, or guilt over sin), and there are other behaviors, sometimes religiously prescribed, which fall within the normal range from the religious viewpoint but not in the light of contemporary psychiatry (e.g., speaking in tongues, prophetic frenzy).

Second, particular types and qualities of religion and levels of religious commitment reflect differently on individuals' psychological needs and types of psychic conflicts. This means that psychological conflict in one religious patient may not always elucidate the religious conflict of another patient who maintains the same religious beliefs. The same holds when comparing the conflicts of converts to new religions, persons who have intensified their commitment to the religion of their childhood, and persons who have maintained a single level of commitment throughout their lives.

Third, a mature religious system may in fact concur with a psychotherapist's judgment of the qualitatively disturbed nature and content of a religious patient's beliefs and practices, and with the need for some modification which will likely include reappraisal of such beliefs and practices, but may at the same time demand that the individual not abandon the basic commitment to the religion or to the rudimentary tenets implicit in even the patient's distorted version of religion. This imposes a constraint upon the mental health worker. Thus, the therapist must be prepared anew with each religious patient to discriminate legitimate from illegitimate uses of religious belief, but also to gauge inter- and intrapersonal imbalance from the perspective of the patient's cultural or ethical background.

Related to the therapist's ability to relate to religious patients with an appropriate balance of professional enthusiasm and detachment is the therapist's ability to monitor and calibrate the unconscious determinants of his own attitudes toward and the need for religion and to prevent these from exerting destructive influence on the clinical alliance with the religious patient. I am speaking about the therapist's understanding of the religious patient's transference responses and the therapist's own unique range of countertransference responses with such patients. While the need to attend to such reactions has been recognized, the literature contains very few papers which discuss how such transference and countertransference manifest and how they are best managed.

Another insufficiently explored area of the therapeutic encounter between the psychotherapist and the religious patient is the specific methodology for dealing with select technical dilemmas which arise in work with such patients. Again, the extant clinical papers offer little by way of precise technique. Examples of these problems are: how the religious patient initially presents his or her problems; initiating discussion with the patient about how the therapist will deal with religion during the course of therapy; consultation with the patient's religious mentors (if recommendable) and the effect of such consultation on confidentiality and preservation of basic trust; the religious patient's idealization of the religious therapist as a religious "mentor"; the relationship between a religious therapist and his religious community; the management of resistances couched in religious or dogmatic attitudinal terms and beliefs; attitudes toward and management of the overall religiosity of psychotic patients; and so forth. The apparent complications posed by issues such as these for the inexperienced therapist motivate some to state in principle that a religious therapist should not undertake treatment of patients of the same religious persuasion. I believe this claim is as nonsensical as barring all male therapists from treating male patients, and so forth. Each of these issues can be dealt with most effectively once one has acquired a certain amount of experience with such patients, and once one establishes some useful and reliable techniques for managing these issues.

It is therefore most important that experienced clinicians who have evolved such techniques be able to present these to other workers. And it is for this reason that the presentation of such experience should be done through the use of many detailed case illustrations which enable the reader to share the writer's experience and to be able to observe exactly how particular problems surface and how they are managed.

The above is a summary of some issues relevant to psychotherapy of the religious patient. Many will be addressed in the forthcoming chapters. It is hoped that the reader will find in these chapters a congenial home for many of his or her own observations, reflections, and management techniques that have proven useful in their own clinical experience. If we have been successful in presenting the forthcoming case illustrations in a manner which allows the material to come alive in the imagination of the reader, then these cases will in a certain sense augment the reader's clinical experience whether or not there is total agreement on the treatment methods utilized.

REFERENCES

Bergin, A. Psychotherapy and religious values. *Journal of Consulting and Clinical Psychology*, 1980, *48*, 95-105.

Casey, R.P. The psychoanalytic study of religion. *Journal of Abnormal and Social Psychology*, 1938, *33*, 437-452.

Cohen, R. & Smith, F. Socially reinforced obsessing: Etiology of a disorder in a Christian Scientist. *Journal of Consulting and Clinical Psychology*, 1976, *44*, 142-144.

Ehrlich, D. & Wiener, D.N. The measurement of values in psychotherapeutic settings. *Journal of Genetic Psychology*, 1961, *64*, 359-372.

Galanter, R., Rabkin, R., Rabkin, J. & Deutsch, A. The "Moonies": A psychological study of conversion and membership in a contemporary religious sect. *American Journal of Psychiatry*, 1979, *136*, 165-170.

Grock, C. On the study of religious commitment. *Religious Education*, 1962, *4*, 98-110.

Halperin, D. (ed.). *Psychodynamic Perspectives on Religion, Sect, and Cult*. Littleton, Mass.: John Wright/P.S.G. Pub., 1983.

Knight, R. Practical and theoretical considerations in the analysis of a minister. *Psychoanalytic Review*, 1937, *24*, 350-364.

Krasner, L. The therapist as a social reinforcement machine. In E.A. Rubenstein & M.B. Parloff (eds.). *Research in Psychotherapy*. Washington, DC: American Psychological Association, 1959.

London, P. *The Modes and Morals of Psychotherapy*. New York: Holt, Rinehart & Winston, 1964.

Mann, J. Clinical and theoretical aspects of religious beliefs. *Journal of the American Psychoanalytical Association*, 1964, *11*, 160-170.

Meehl, P. Some technical and axiological problems in the therapeutic handling of religious and valuational material. *Journal of Consulting Psychology*, 1959, *6*, 255-259.

Pattison, E.M. The development of ego morality. *Psychoanalytic Review*, 1968, *55*, 187-222.

Pattison, E.M. Psychiatry and religion circa 1978: Analysis of a decade, Part I. *Pastoral Psychology*, 1978, *27*, 8-25. (a)

Pattison, E.M. Psychiatry and religion circa 1978: Analysis of a decade, Part II. *Pastoral Psychology*, 1978, *27*, 119-141. (b)

Pattison, E.M. Religious youth cults: Alternative healing social networks. *Journal of Religion and Health*, 1980, *19*, 275-286.

Pruyser, P. The seamy side of current religious beliefs. *Bulletin of the Menninger Clinic*, 1977, *41*, 329-340.

Rizzuto, A.M. *The Birth of a Living God: A Psychoanalytic Study*. Chicago: University of Chicago Press, 1979.

Rizzuto, A.M. Object-relations and the formation of the image of God. *British Journal of Medical Psychology*, 1974, *47*, 83-99.

Shapiro, E. Destructive cults. *American Family Physician*, 1977, *15*, 80-83.

Spero, M.H. *Judaism and Psychology: Halakhic Perspectives.* New York: Ktav/Yeshiva University Press, 1980.

Spero, M.H. Psychotherapeutic procedure with religious cult devotees. *Journal of Nervous and Mental Disease*, 1982, *170*, 332-344.

Stark, R. Psychopathology and religious commitment. *Review of Religious Research*, 1971, *12*, 165-175.

Wile, P. Ideological conflict between therapist and patient. *American Journal of Psychotherapy*, 1977, *31*, 437-449.

Wolberg, L.R. *The Technique of Psychotherapy.* New York: Grune & Stratton, 1977.

Section Two
DIAGNOSIS AND ASSESSMENT

Chapter 2

DIAGNOSTIC GUIDELINES FOR PSYCHOTHERAPY OF THE RELIGIOUS PATIENT

MOSHE HALEVI SPERO, Ph.D.

THE following chapter presents a schematic of diagnostic characteristics for discriminating autonomous from dysautonomous or "pathologic" religious belief and behavior. Some basic treatment principles and procedures will also be outlined. In a final section I will illustrate the emergence of disordered religiosity during the psychological testing process, and attempt to distinguish these manifestations from other test behaviors that could be considered normative for the subgroup of religious patients. The support body from which these guidelines have been distilled is amply represented in the chapters contained in this text, although I will include in the following section some representative case illustrations from my clinical experience with orthodox Jewish clientele.

DIAGNOSTIC CHARACTERISTICS

In diagnosing the patient with maladaptive religious beliefs and practices, the clinician must consider foremost that the patient's religious values are not extraneous to the therapeutic scope, but rather are a potential playground for narcissistic, libidinal, and aggressive drives and tendencies, and are readily co-opted in the service of the ego by neurotic organizing processes. Second, religious systems, normal or otherwise, can influence the overall course of psychological development, producing specific and characteristic types of strengths or impairments or simply unique qualities in the levels of ego functioning. Like all ego adaptations to inner and outer reality, religious belief can take either autonomous or dysautonomous forms, indicative of normal as well as neurotic perceptions and modes of adjustment, and can manifest itself in any of the various ego functions, such as reality-testing, defense functioning, sense of mastery-competence, judgment, object-relations, and so forth. These dynamic axia also apply to the psychotherapist's religious beliefs or lack of them.

One approach to assessing psychopathology in religious personalities is to highlight key problem areas typical of this subgroup. Sevensky (1984) discusses eight areas of therapeutic focus with religious patients: (1) the "weak faith" syndrome, (2) the demand for a therapist of the same faith, (3) the search for magical cure, (4) religious idealization and identification, (5) demonic possession, (6) the inability to feel forgiven, (7) the feeling that one has been abandoned by God, and (8) other areas of potential pyschopathology such as glossalalia, conversion, etc.

Perhaps a diagnostically-focused approach would be more useful for most dynamically oriented practitioners. The inference that disordered psychological need or conflict underlies a particular patient's religious belief or behavior is best made in the presence of the following characteristics (see Pruyser, 1976, 1977; Spero, 1980).

(1) The individual expresses religious behaviors and beliefs that are somehow related to overall lifestyle. This characteristic is itself not necessarily pathologic, but is necessary as a basic criterion.

(2) The individual's total religious affiliation, or the current intensity or sense of religious meaning and conviction, is of relatively recent and rapid onset and has involved the individual in severing one or more significant family, social, or professional ties and roles.

(3) The individual's past history includes numerous religious

"crises" or episodes of changing religious affiliations or levels of belief.

(4) The individual's religious behaviors and beliefs evince fixation at or regression to specific clusters of object-relational pathology, typified by (a) the predominace of primitive object-relational thematic material in dream, fantasy, or thought productions which are unarticulated with developmentally appropriate psychosexual or object-relational themes, (b) lack of integration between the individual's mode of religious expression and adaptive ego functioning, and (c) failure to successfully accomplish appropriate psychosocial tasks (see also Draper, *et al*, 1965).

Typical clusters which highlight inappropriate balance between religiosity and psychosocial development are:

  (i) Oral-narcissistic religion; e.g., the search for narcissistic satisfaction through group identification or attitudes toward God; hypercathexis of the self and concomitant withdrawal of interest in healthy interpersonal relations; passivity; manipulation of others in the interests of self-satisfaction; hypomanic, childlike investment in repetitive ritual enactments; grandiose ideation.

  (ii) Anal religiosity; e.g., passive-aggressive noncompliance with parental norms or social norms; neurotic shame and self-hate; the adoption of monastic rigor in partial fulfillment of the need to be vilified; inappropriate and unconstructive humility and self-negation; obsessive preoccupation with right and wrong, sin, guilt, scrupulosity, etc.

  (iii) Phallic and oedipal religiosity; e.g., conflicts surrounding mastery-competence, curiosity, pride, competition, sexual relations, adolescent rebellion, guilt, etc. In some cases, "phallic" and "oedipal" preoccupations ensconced in religious-like behaviors or attitudes can mask anxiety-provoking disturbances at earlier levels of development, such as borderline disturbances or gender confusion.

(5) The religious individual is preoccupied either with a directly acknowledged or intellectually masked fear of back-sliding and the reactive adoption of rigidity, scrupulosity, and puncti-

liousness in the attempt to deal with such fears. This is sometimes manifest in the adoption of strict interpretations of religious law when the prevailing custom follows a lenient
interpretation *and* where there is obvious discomfort with
adopting lenient interpretations.

(6) Continued unhappiness and improductivity following religious conversion or awakening.

(7) Excessive idealization of a religious movement or leader, and
the use of such idealization to resolve problems of autonomy,
identity, impulse control, and so forth.

(8) Occasionally, the cautiously interpreted countertransference
reaction of a well-analyzed and experienced worker can also
serve as a minimal indicator of the patient's attempt to use religion as a tool to satisfy neurotic needs.

Rizzuto (1979, pp. 206-207) illustrates the many levels of relationship between psychosocial and psychodynamic functioning and
development and the representation of God and religious experience. She emphasizes in particular the complementarity between
persons' God concepts and object concepts at each stage of life.
While her approach depicts a developmental progression, it is always possible that an individual who has achieved some higher level
of functioning or representation may regress to more primitive
levels, such as during the initial stages of conversion or as a result of
affiliation with pathological religions such as cults. Second, just as
the quality of individuals' psychosexual development and achieve-
ments in self-other differentiation influences their perception and
experience of God and spirituality, so do parental and environmen-
tal models of religiosity and divinity — and the potential for transference between attitudes toward God and parents — influence
individuals' perception of parents, peers, self, and environment.
This will be evident within the transferences which occur throughout
the lifetime as well as during psychotherapy.

Guntrip provides an illuminating example of this point (1969, p.
351). He records a patient's dream:

I'm looking for Christ on the seashore. He rose up as if out of the
sea and I admired his tall, magnificent figure. Then I went with

Him to a cave and became conscious of ghosts there and fled in
stark terror. But He stayed and I mustered up the courage and
went back in with Him. Then the cave was a house, as He and I
went upstairs, He said, "You proved to have greater courage than
I had," and I felt I detected some weakness in Him.

The patient's subsequent associations included a comparison between his admiration for both Christ's and his own father's athletic
figures, and then with the therapist's. "I also associate Him with you.
I've got the idea that somehow you may inveigle me into courage to
face ghosts and then let me down. Mother was a menacing figure.
Father was weak, mute before her onslaughts. He once said it wasn't
a good thing to have one parent constantly dominating the other in
front of a child, but he never showed any anger at all."

Guntrip suggest that the patient oscillated between an old fear
that the father let the patient down if he tried to stand up to his violently tempered mother, and a new wavering hope that the therapist
would not let him down as he prepared to confront the "ghost" or image of the angry mother. The therapist was being gradually internalized as a reliable parent-figure, and was given divine, savior-like
characteristics. Doubtless, the patient's image and experience of
God was colored by the same sense of disappointment or anger for
previous let downs and perhaps the hope of future strength. What is
most important is that the human object relationship influences the
divine object relationship and *vice versa*. These mutual and compli-
mentary influences can be expected to show up in individual's attitudes toward prayer, God's role in the evil in the world, repentance
and reward and punishment, and so forth. It thus can be no less anticipated that patients who are frustrated with or angry at their God
will in the course of transference in therapy demonstrate similar attitudes toward the therapist, and even attempt to replace God with the
image of the therapist.

As mentioned above, in the case of individuals currently undergoing religious crisis, such as the convert or the penitent personality,
some of the above characteristics may be evident as an outcome of
the *gradual process* of breaking with and resolving past ties and identifications and consolidating new ones, and of adapting to new ways
of life or new perceptions which require the devaluing of former
ways and the restriction of formerly unrestricted ego and instinctual

expressions. Furthermore, in the process of conversion or radical in-
creases in religiosity, the crucial trauma or crisis is not simply the
abandonment of secular attitudes or other familiar habits and beliefs
and the adoption of new beliefs or rituals, but moreso the transformations in narcissism and reworking of object-relationships that will
have to ensue. Some "rebelliousness" is necessary for the achievement of separation from former ways or ties and the adoption of new
ways of life, some increased investment in the self is necessary to off-
set the libidinal losses resulting from broken ties and criticisms of
others, some reaction-formation can be expected in the process of re-
nunciating old channels and modes of sexual and aggressive expression, and so forth. Yet, these temporary qualities during the process
of religious change always represent potential for both creative
growth or fixation and regression, and must be monitored carefully
to prevent the recrudescence of unresolved psychosexual or psychosocial conflicts which may lead to the adoption of pathologic religious expressions as ends in themselves.

This diagnostic outline does not imply that *normal* religion is
merely the absence or reverse of these characteristics, or that normal
religion cannot transcend these infantile qualities. It is intended primarily as a shorthand of one approach to detecting evidence of dysautonomous religiosity, highlighting pathologic characteristics in
terms that can be immediately translated into practice by a wide variety of mental health professionals (see Bibliography).

CASE ILLUSTRATIONS

Patients who maintain dysautonomous religious beliefs often
evince religious-like attention to the consensual values and practices
of normal religion, but which in fact caricaturize autonomous religious practice. At the same time, the patient who considers himself
authentically religious may be only dimly aware of any unevenness
or peculiarity in his religiosity. The clinician must respond to both
the neurotic and valid or authentic religious aspects of such personalities and assess their qualities in terms of the characteristics discussed in this chapter. The following case studies will illustrate some
dysautonomous qualities of religious behavior.

CASE 1: MAX

Max, a lawyer, bacame intensely religious at age 23 and married a "modern orthodox" Jewish girl from a religious family. A fairly intelligent individual, Max progressively integrated the demands of religious practice and belief in what seemed initially to be an appropriate manner. Friends of the wife's family, however, frequently remarked that Max was becoming a bit "square," and perhaps too willing to accept doctrinaire beliefs without subjecting these beliefs to the type of sharp scrutiny typical of Max's earlier levels of religious growth. Max soon surpassed the religious level of his wife's family and circle and, in relocating to accept a new professional appointment, came into company of a supportive yet fundamentalisitc Jewish religious group. Needing to assimilate yet another, more rigid approach to Jewish values as a substitute for his increasing loss of early childhood and adolescent relationships and identifications, Max's ardent Zionism gave way to a fundamentalistic belief in the intrinsic value of living in Diaspora: style of clothing and dogmatic group beliefs became central concerns; and he began to question the religious value of his own secular involvements and professional role. It was not long before Max was supined by efforts spent on perfecting ritual according to minority opinion requirements, purchasing costly volumes of Jewish law which he could not yet comprehend, naively accepting the latest in-group myths and political opinions, purchasing an additional pair of phylacteries and another *talit* just in case his original sets *might* become ritually unfit, and getting involved in heated quasi-philosophical debate at the slightest challenge.

Max's apprehensions and doubts had no basis in any normative approach to Jewish practice and belief. Max had fixated at a stage where the possibility of religious backsliding and the pressure to conform so as to gain entrance into a significant social group compromised the need for individuality. Following the advice of the author, whose opinion was sought by a concerned friend and religious teacher, Max was helped to understand and confront the emotional strain he was experiencing by severing so many family ties, his fears of not being accepted, and his shame and guilt over his family's religious ignorance and his own irreligious childhood and adolescence.

Max initially denied these carefully administered interpretations, but it was possible to point out to him the discomfort he experienced when discussing his past relationships and views as well as his idealization of certain religious leaders and acquaintances with whom, despite their religious collegiality, he truly did not get along. As Max became more comfortable with maintaining his family ties he experienced a lessened need to deny his unrecognized ambivalence toward his early lifestyle as well as to the dogmatic religious ways of his current social group. Max broadened his religious affiliations and began to ease comfortably into a more appropriate level of religious observance commensurate with his realistic needs, his emotional preparedness, and his gradually increasing sense of religious growth. While Max currently retains some of the later-adopted religious beliefs and practices, they have become integrated with an appropriate sense of individuality, a more critical attitude, and with less of the pressure to conform.

CASE 2: NAHSHON

Nahshon, age 20, was raised in a reform Jewish environment, and was dominated by an authoritarian father who exerted extreme pressure on Nahshon to continue a family heritage in the medical profession. Nahshon was an anxious and fearful individual, riddled by self-doubt and given to rebellious fantasies as a sole means of escaping the pressuring atmosphere of home life. Nahshon envisioned his startling announcement of electing ecological studies as a college major as an assertion of his individualism, but this choice only increased tensions and difficulties with his family.

During his freshman year, Nahshon was influenced by the Moon cult and paradoxically claimed to experience a sense of "fulfillment" through the intense, "pressure free" comaraderie among the cult members. This sense of freedom was actually the result of adopting a highly polarized way of life where anti-parental tendencies were given normative status. Nahshon was rising in the ranks of this group to a position of long-desired leadership—a parental disenthronement—when his parents managed to secret him out of the group and had him deprogrammed. Nahshon initially appeared relieved at regaining his freedom, though he was uncharacteristically taciturn and depressed. He shortly resumed college courses. During the subsequent months — critical for meaningfully filling the spiritual and psychological vacuum that occurs in the wake of the sense of loss many individuals experience after being deprogrammed (Spero, 1983) — Nahshon became attracted to the local campus Hasidic Jewish group. Though not in any way cultlike in style or intent, the Hasidic group also tended to stress peripheral ritualistic activities and pleasurable sensations as one way to interest "errant" or unknowledgable Jews to return to the fold. For many individuals who embark upon a similar path with such groups, this initial stage of childlike mystification and also vulnerability eventually develops into a more intellectually and personally satisfying commitment. Nahshon's new religious phase soon developed into frenzied involvement in dancing, style of clothing, laughing at in-group jokes or listening blankly to in-group stories, and minimal prayer behavior. Nahshon was now prepared to accept that matters spiritual preceded in importance all other earthly concerns. Yet, his religious developments were not deepening in an integrated or meaningful way. Again he dropped out of college, despite the protests of his new religious leader.

Once he decided to commit himself to learning Torah and Jewish studies, the religious leader had no choice but to acknowledge that this was a lofty and valuable goal, even though he told Nahshon that he was not yet completely ready for total immersion into the new life-style that these studies would require. At the same time, Nahshon's decision exacerbated his family conflicts. The solace Nahshon had earlier derived from his affiliation with the Hasidic group now turned into a bitter struggle as he demanded of the group and its rabbi the "right" to their support against his family's pleas. Constant bickering occured over trivial issues. Nahshon renounced this reli-

gious group in the same precipitious way he joined it, and on the advice of friends, dropped from its circles and resumed his college
courses, changing his major to pre-medicine. He was repulsed by
any attempts to win him back into the Hasidic group. Two months
following his break with this religious group, Nahshon moved away
from home and joined a therapeutically-oriented communal group
in California.

CASE 3: SARA

I have recently reported in detail the case of Sara, a young,
orthodox Jewish wife accepted into psychoanalytic treatment. An
hysterical personality in the classic sense, Sara presented with a
unique symptom of functional irregular uterine cramping and
bleeding. This young woman was very narcissistic and, in addition
to highly conflicted oedipal strivings and hostilities, suffered from an
early childhood and adolescent upbringing in the emotionally confusing atmosphere produced by parents who were concentration
camp survivors. Unable to deal with their own depression and mor-
bid preoccupations, Sara's parents provided her with a confusing relationship to a hysterical mother and an emotionally-withdrawn
father. The traumatic memory of witnessing the unfortunate mis-
handling of her mother's miscarriage also had a disorganizing effect
on her attitudes toward femininity and sexuality in general. This patient was able to carry out an effective denial of sexuality and an unconscious destruction of her parents through her symptom, which,
reinforced by scrupulous observance of Jewish laws of family purity
(which required the frequent suspension of physical contact with her
husband because of her menstrual status), enabled her to replicate in
her own married life the cold and emotionally negative atmosphere
of her childhood.

Eventually successful psychotherapy was achieved by accepting
the patient's religious beliefs and expressed attitude toward sexuality
but working around them to uncover the disorganized emotional
needs expressed through such beliefs. The therapist did not require
the patient to renounce her religious convictions, but rather confronted the narcissistic and aggressive trends that emerged within

therapy as Sara attempted to manipulate this encounter in characteristic ways. Tolerance of her slowly increasing ability to express
emotional confusion, grief, and a deep sense of unjust parental treatment, enabled her to pull away fron the guilt-reinforced retaliation
cycle. From this stage, Sara was able to reconsider her earlier attitudes toward sexuality and to successfully differentiate her hated
God-father and God-mother introjects. At this stage, the patient experienced symptom relief and progressed toward a more mature
feminine sexual identification.

The following case illustrates the influence of shame dynamics
upon religious growth. I have included this brief vignette because of
the frequency with which I have encountered shame-oriented
dynamics in the penitent religious personality.

CASE 4: EARL

Earl, a 20 year-old, became orthodox at the age of 19. His initial
interest in orthodox Judaism emerged coincidental with similar developments in a best friend with whom Earl operated a summer
business. Earl's friend became intensely attached to a naive, blissful
interpretation of Judaism, but soon became increasingly irrealistic,
eventually suffering an acute psychotic episode during which he
imagined himself to be Messiah. Following emergency psychiatric
treatment and subsequent psychotherapy, the friend discarded his
orthodoxy, moving back to his original level of minimal commitment
and practice. Earl initially experienced a reaction against his own religious strivings following his friend's unfortunate regression, and
also pulled away from their formerly close relationship. Subsequently, however, Earl began to move forward in religious interest at
a reasonable and cautious pace.

Within a year, Earl took temporary leave of absence from college
studies and went to Israel where he engaged in religious study at a
well-known yeshiva. Within this interval, Earl made considerable
gains in religious knowledge and observance, adopting more or less
typical orthodox Jewish attitudes, habits, and demeanor. Though
there were apparently many autonomous aspects to Earl's religious
development, evidence of conflict was never far from the surface.

Like many of his cohorts undergoing similar crises, Earl rapidly idealized his religious teachers. More significantly, Earl remained lonely, lacked a clear sense of direction, and found it difficult to relate to his peers. By the end of the year, Earl decided to return to America.

Once back home, situated in a highly orthodox Jewish community, Earl's anomie, lack of direction, and insecurity increased. He began to experience gnawing doubts about his previous interest in and intensity of religious commitment, feeling "abandoned" by earlier religious acquaintances who initially brought him closer to Judaism who now either had insufficient time for him or, as Earl perceived it, looked down upon his return to America and his ambivalence about continuing yeshiva education at the local yeshiva — or were too old or too young to satisfy the need to replace his former irreligious comrades with a new set of religious friends. Throughout, Earl's parents were supportive, though they expressed open concern about his intense commitment, frequently reminding him of earlier fadistic and equally intense commitments in his past.

Earl freely elected psychotherapy in order to deal with unaccountable tiredness and poor health (headaches, sleeplessness, colds), indecision regarding continuing college, loneliness, and the reappearance of obsessive worrying trends. He noted that he had brief psychotherapeutic experiences in the past, but that these never provided long-term improvement. Earl eventually added that many of his fears and insecurities extended back to earliest school years. He also recalled that as a child he had many tics and was always an "overachiever." In early weeks of therapy, Earl ruminated about decision-making problems, fears of "sinful" sexual impulses when meeting girls, fears of meeting old friends and establishing new ones, and worried about being thought of as a "sissy" or "flipped out." Yet to be expressed during initial sessions was the anxiety associated with having become that which in his youth he himself would have considered "queer," or otherwise devalued (a frequent problem of the adolescent *ba'al teshuvah* who, by becoming more religious, thereby fulfills a negative image he may have held toward orthodox Jews).

The therapist's refusal to give advice and religious interpretations to pseudoreligious questions ("Should I go to yeshiva?" "Can I look at girls when I'm in college?" "How many hours should I spend on

Talmud studies?"), and the therapist's insistance that these sorts of questions be explored from within the overall therapeutic focus, initially irritated Earl's narcissistic-demanding trends, but eventually promoted the return of healthy self-acceptance, mature decision-making, and also prevented Earl from idealizing the therapist. Many of these demands were eventually understood as religiously-couched expressions of transference wherein the therapist would be transformed into the critical, perfectionistic, and obsessive father-figure, only who would now be utilized as a "religious" superego ideal as opposed to the shaming superego ideals of Earl's youth. The fear of failure and the impunitive reactions to perceived or fantasied imperfection in Earl's new way of life were essentially not much different than the fears and self-debasing tendencies which characterized his early years. The therapist also explored with Earl his fears about being "crazy," especially in the light of Earl's own perception of his friend's "religious" crisis. Eventually, Earl was able to narrow his associations and focus on his deeper doubts about himself, and began to relate more productively to his family and intrapersonal problems. These included a painful sense of distance from his father who had himself been orthodox in his earliest years though currently uncommitted, and who also suffered from some manic-depressive disorder, and a deep sense of inadequacy and shame. Many of Earl's oedipal conflicts and shame-proneness were apparently disguised behind the search for superego replacements which would offer much needed supplies in his chosen, new area of competence—his religious devotion—and which were now failing him. Earl's own insecurity about his leveling-off in religious intensity since his return from Israel (though not in the area of practice and basic commitment) added the anxiety that he was failing in this new area as well.

He eventually recovered a traumatic memory from his toilet-training years in which his mother had smeared his face with feces because the patient was being stubborn and noncompliant. He was eventually able to accept that his dissatisfaction with all of his life goals and efforts, including his new religiosity, was essentially the result of an intensely neurotic perfectionism designed to prevent all shame and incompetence, and to appease hateful maternal and paternal introjects. The patient's shame over his own religious behaviors, such as wearing his skullcap in public, was rooted in recurrent fantasies that these new customs attracted attention to his "shit-smeared face."

Thus, though much of Earl's loneliness and anomie was realistic given the major changes he had undergone in communal and interpersonal affiliation and interest, a significant portion of these disturbing feelings stemmed from much more deeply-rooted object-relational deficits. His alternating feelings of being isolated from or hated by the Jewish community *versus* feeling smothered by the community's overinvestment in his personal growth, and similar vascilations in his feelings toward God, were largely determined by poor self-other differentiation resulting from so many early experiences with shaming, intrusive introjects. From this perspective, conflict in overall religious growth persisted to the degree that Earl's religious development represented a neurotic attempt to escape shaming introjects and to replace these with all-providing, all-rewarding internal objects, divine and human. His hesitancy in social relationships could now be understood in terms of hiding shameful aspects of himself from others, and his interest in Judaism could be seen as containing elements of an attempt at mastery over others as well as for himself. The patient's disordered uses and misinterpretations of religion were resolved by submitting religious as well as general issues to standard psychoanalytic techniques of free association and interpretation, and helping the patient to explore fully each aspect of his religious life. Very often, apparently religious material led to important dynamic associations, and what seemed like general issues led to associations colored with religious references which in turn led to conplex dynamic issues. Earl was soon able to surrender the idealized substitutes he had adopted to resolve this search, and to restructure his personality so that his interest in Judaism could be liberated from long-standing conflicts. The mastery he truly sought could now be achieved.

CASE 5: ROBERT

A most interesting combination of distorted and healthy religious strivings enmeshed in family and intrapersonal dynamics occured in a 17 year-old Jewish high school student. Robert came from a modern orthodox Jewish family and attended an orthodox high school. His father was a successful entrepeneur and his mother was a housewife, both of whom were survivors of the Nazi extermination camps. The patient was the youngest sibling of four sisters. He was socially active and academically successful. Psychotherapy was initiated for Robert by the parents following an incident where he had tearfully admitted going to women's clothing stores and trying on women's undergarments in the dressing room. During the initial consult, Robert added that on an earlier occasion two years prior to therapy he had exhibited himself in the presence of some neighborhood girls, and that he had a compulsion to call up clothing stores and ask the saleslady if her store stocked leotards, brassiers, and so forth. The patient was very bothered about these behaviors and about his inability to control them. He mentioned that he had undergone a brief half-year period of intense religiosity when he was 14 years old during which time he prayed desperately for God's help, but this apparently did not help. He also had seen another psychologist for about one year, but "aside from a lot of the therapist's talking," Robert felt he had accomplished nothing. I offered him psychoanalysis with sessions thrice-weekly.

Further exploration of Robert's symptom revealed that prior to each incident of calling or going to stores, or occasionally purchasing pornographic magazines, he would enter a state of listlessness and boredom. No matter how strenuously he argued with himself at other times about the degrading, religiously vile, and possibly unlawful nature of these behaviors, once he entered his "boredom" state he could think about nothing else save carrying through his impulse. He also explained that he felt a certain calming feeling as he would converse with the salesladies; preferring young salesladies to "older sounding women" to the degree that if an older woman answered the phone, he would hang up. The exhibiting behavior occurred only twice, and he felt embarrassed enough never to repeat this behavior, although he recalled that he had felt "good" and then "silly and foolish" as he watched the stunned reactions of his audience.

Robert was generally a willing and able subject for psychoanalytic treatment despite expectable adolescent and other forms of resistance. He demonstrated a gradual disinterest in making calls or visiting stores after the first five months of treatment. Summer vacation became an issue at this point, and I strongly urged that we continue our work. The father intruded at this point and, satisfied with Robert's success to this point, arranged for an extended trip for the patient. During the hiatus, Robert felt compelled to try on some women's clothes at a department store and was apprehended by the house detective. The patient and his father called me in panic and asked me to intervene. The detective was most understanding and dropped charges so long as the young man continued in therapy. Following this crisis, which was partly motivated by Robert's desire to get back into therapy, Robert continued in analysis for another two years at which point he and the therapist agreed that he was prepared for a year of college abroad. There were only four incidents of telephone calls to stores subsequent to angry fights with his father during the first seven months of this second stage of therapy, and none following.

Several topics emerged during the psychoanalysis. One had to do with the influence of his older sisters and their penchant for babying him and dressing him as a girl or a clown during his early childhood. He recalled feeling unable to do much about this at such a young age, yet enjoying the attention of others. Subsequent analysis uncovered the deep shame and resentment he experienced during these episodes.

A second, major topic centered upon his parents' physical, psychological, and religious status. Both parents had serious physical systemic illnesses requiring at least one major surgery for both and a host of real and hypochondriachal complaints and preoccupations at home. Either one or both of the parents seemed to Robert to be forever groaning, collapsing, threatening death or debilitation. Often, the parents, but primarily the father, linked their ailments to the patient's behavior, such as not achieving straight A's, not being serious enough about his religious studies, not praying with a fervor commensurate with a deeply *"yeshivasheh"* (yeshiva-like) attitude, and so forth. Yet, throughout the early period of therapy, Robert denied the possibility that his parents' death anxiety and frequent illness had any great impact upon him, saying, "If you grow up with it, I guess it doesn't really shock you." The patient adopted the same defensive attitude regarding his parents' open bathroom door policy, speaking in a rather blasé fashion about the sights and smells he had grown accustomed to during his childhood and early adolescence (at which point the first psychologist had instructed the parents to discontinue this policy). Interpretation at this point of Robert's lapses into boredom preceeding his calls showed that this state served to deny anger and other feelings, and also to short circuit his sense of judgment and thinking processes, thereby allowing his symptomatic behavior more ready expression.

A third theme focused around the father's dramatic, boastful manner, which applied to everything from his acts of charity, his life style, his survival of Hitler, his return to orthodoxy following several post-war years of angry disbelief (discussed below), his son's academic accomplishment, to his powerful friends in positions of influence, and so forth. Father was indeed a good and kindly person, but was also experienced by Robert as relentlessly demanding, perfectionistic, pigheaded, argumentative, and as operating with perplexing double standards and contradictory demands.

The most significant domain of double standard in the father's behavior was religiosity. Robert consciously admired his father's return to faith, but also felt intolerable his father's refusal to acknowledge the similarities between his own period of doubt and the patient's, the patient's friends' and their families' religious weaknesses and his father's own, and the father's frequent disdainful tales of the oppressive atmosphere of his childhood religious environment and the one he was presently creating in Robert's life. He recounted how his father would badger him about the need to be deeply religious — which Robert always felt was directed more at appearances rather than truly authentic religiosity, which he felt he would surely "grow into" if his father would just let him develop normally — and then father would be caught "stealing a smoke in the bathroom on Shabbat" or turning on a light on Shabbat. The father admitted that he still had his areas of weakness, but the patient felt that no such allowance was made for him.

The course of self-exploration during analysis was often impeded by the father's attempts to use the analyst as an extension of his own educational and moral influence, and by more than once holding forth the contradictory wish that the analyst help him to accept his son more realistically and that the analyst more quickly admonish the patient to heed his father's demands and perspectives. However, I was successful in parying this influence and, with the patient's permission, scheduled a few joint sessions, and some additional ones solely with the father, which enabled me at least to achieve the father's respect for his son's privacy and individuality as well as a not small amount of self-understanding and maturity on the father's part.

Our therapeutic work revealed that the patient's symptoms and other identity-related and minor religious doubts expressed, on different but multidetermined levels, a way to deny castration and death anxiety through the mechanism of protesting his masculinity and his ability to shock women. The display behavior was both a reaction against a shame-ridden core as well as a dramatization of his ambivalence toward his father's "showiness" and his attempts to display his only son. The patient discovered the sense in which his feeling for the unknown woman on the other end of the telephone satisfied an intense fear of object loss and loss of love.

One particular incident helped bring this last insight to the fore. During Robert's last call to a store, he had asked a saleslady for leotards, telling her he was living with a mean aunt (probably a displacement of his sisters' imago) who forced him to dress as a lady when he misbehaved. The saleslady appeared to be sincerely upset that he allowed himself to be so treated. She told him that he should not obey her and also get himself some help with this. The patient was taken aback, mumbled his appreciation to the woman, and hung up. Subsequent associations to this produced a memory of Robert as a terrified 5 year-old youngster desperately searching for his mother who had told him to wait for her by a doctor's office and then, without telling him, had gone for a moment to another doctor's office. The patient recalled that they were quickly reunited, but he was inconsolate for a few hours that day. He then spoke of his feeling that parents cannot truly love a child if they claim they love the child but intend to leave the child, or die! He connected these thoughts with feeling that h is parents had left h im with a sense of their impermanence and did nothing to reassure him of the opposite. The saleslady on the phone, he now believed, had at least been honest enough to tell him that things were not as he said they were.

A great deal of analytic focus was directed to Robert's image of and feelings toward God. As could be expected, the patient experienced God in the same fashion as he experienced his father, and to a degree his mother: arbitrary, demanding, contradictory ("He asks that we do his commandments, but Jews still get persecuted...and *Moshiach* [Messiah] still hasn't come!"), and not demonstrating love. Although the patient at no time stopped performing religious commandments, and continued to excell in his talmudic studies, his religious behavior was motivated by rote. I did not attempt directly to ordain what level of religious feeling or attitude toward God the patient ought to develop. However, as he developed greater understanding for his father's own problems and differentiated himself from the fears and needs projected upon him by his parents, Robert was able to experience God as a being whom he simply did not yet know or understand. That is, he recognized as merely transfered those hostile and indifferent feelings he displaced onto God and that he truly had no deep convictions about God's inherent badness or indifference. From this vantage point, he was now able to appreciate how others were able to maintain positive, loving attitudes toward God despite the various historical and personal troubles he earlier felt "proved" his negative characterization of God. The patient became more interested and intellectually invested in religious Zionism, and to spend some time studying in a yeshiva in Israel, all of which appeared to express the beginning of a warmer relationship with God and Judaism.

THREE INTERVENTIVE PRINCIPLES

Three basic practice principles must guide psychotherapeutic treatment of patients with both psychological and religious disorder. First, the clinician must gauge the degree of autonomy with which the ego responds to the constructive, growth-provoking aspects of religious belief, the degree to which conflict and secondary autonomous pathologic behaviors are expressed through religious belief and practice, and the ways in which religious belief is used as a resistance to progress in psychotherapy. This approach is similar to the standard therapeutic focus on the ways speech, cognitive, defense, affective, and other ego functions in general are incorporated by neurotic or more primitive organizing processes. The psychotherapist's target is religiosity which masks rather than transcends the infantile and which provides a form of regression and stagnation thinly disguised by behaviors or beliefs which are only superficially religious. Such forms of religion have a rigid quality and are determined by and perpetuate neuroteogenic forces in personality which typically indicate fixation at earlier modes of psychosexual and psychosocial development. This will be obvious both in the manifest qualities of the patient's religiosity as well as in the particular types of "religious" resistances which are likely to occur throughout psychotherapy.

Second, the patient's religious beliefs, ideals, and practices must be subjected to the same nonjudgmental analysis and exploration as are all other aspects of personality, not only in the effort to determine their relative autonomy from pathologic determinants, but also to lessen their utility for the patient as a source of magical hope, denial, or other resistances. At the same time, the therapist does not randomly select isolated religious practices or ideas as targets for criticism or for the imposition of his preconceptions, but rather encourages the patient to express himself freely and completely and to integrate the analytic, self-reflective process. The patient can then take his own religious expressions as objects of this focus, examining them in light of his own deeply-felt psychosocial crises, presenting compliants, and the insights he begins to acquire during therapy.

During the initial encounter with the religious patient or family during the assessment stage, the following kinds of questions need to be addressed (some of which are drawn from Krasner, 1981-21, p. 113-114). From the standpoint of the patient's history and material produced during therapy, one investigates:

1. What are his or her criteria of religion?
2. What are the sources of his criteria: parents, grandparents, mate, clergy, peers?
3. Where and how do people's religious expectations of the patient collide?
4. How does he handle colliding religious expectations?
5. What religious convictions, if any, has he chosen for himself?
6. What is the function and goal of religion in his life?
7. Does religion serve to modify his behavior? How?
8. Is religion a source of friction in his family of origin? In his nuclear family? Is it a source of harmony?
9. What difference does religion make?
10. Is religious observance a resource to family members, or is it a source of conflict?
11. Is religious ritual forced to do the work of relationship for him or her; that is, does it function in lieu of candor and intimacy?
12. Is there room for differing expressions of religious observance in the family? To what degree?
13. How are differences in the person's family negotiated and resolved?
14. Do his or her religious attitudes and behavior in family of procreation force him into disloyalty to his family of origin?
15. How have parental differences over religion forced the person into a situation of split loyalties?
16. Do religious texts, guidelines, rituals, holidays, liturgy and prayer:
    a. Free the person or bind him?
    b. Enable fair give-and-take or restrict it?
    c. Contribute to openness and flexibility or to defensiveness and rigidity?
    d. Make him judgmental or receptive to other people's views?
    e. Help the person address and handle shame and guilt or drive him deeper into it?
    f. Underwrite compulsive tendencies or prod him to new growth?
    g. Help actualize forgiveness or provide a leverage for blame?

    h. Encourage responsibility or its abandonment to others?
17. If the patient is newly religious, what potential conflicts exist between his former and current lifestyle, beliefs, and attitudes? What is his or her sense of the past and how is it expressed and dealt with? What ideals, attitudes, and goals — fantasy or real — has the individual felt obligated to surrender? I have often seen that toward the "middle-life" of such persons' religious living, after the belated newness of their religious feelings has diminished, a conflict emerges between current religious self-images and ideals and the reactivated attractiveness of previously surrendered ideals.
18. Is the patient likely to use the therapist as an alternate "religious" object or need-satisfying ideal?

From the standpoint of the therapist's personal history and reactions during therapy with such patients, one investigates:

1. Do religious references and language from a patient evoke ambivalence of anxiety in a clinician?
2. To what degree has a clinician resolved his own religious conflicts so that he can more readily distinguish the terms of his patient's context from that of his own?
3. To what degree are a patient's religious loyalties, his synagogue, his rabbi or priest, ritual, and meditation or prayer a resource to the clinican?
4. Does a patient's investment in God accord with his clinician's criteria for mental health?
5. Does the therapist experience particular difficulties with certain kinds of religious belief or levels of religious belief?
6. What kind of transference and countertransference can be anticipated in view of the particular way the patient is likely to experience the therapist's personality, religiosity, and interventions?

Throughout, the definition of "relative autonomy" of religious experience remains the patient's to the degree that it approximates the true perspectives of the particular religious system involved (assuming that it is not itself a destructive religious system such as cults). This is necessarily a constraint on the therapeutic goals which can be achieved with a particular patient. That is, the therapeutic goal with a religious patient is not the removal of his essential commitment to religion, or his basic obligation to religious practice, but aiding him to achieve a less conflicted state of belief. If the patient perceives himself as religious, then the therapist aids the patient to experience religion in an adaptive fashion.

TRANSFERENCE — COUNTERTRANSFERENCE

The third practice principle relates to the management of transference and countertransference reactions. The religious therapist must monitor his own religious feelings, or lack of them, and be cognizant of the potential in such an encounter for negative as well as positive attitudes to emerge which can distort the therapeutic alliance. The potentially destructive impact in the therapeutic alliance of anti-religious bias and even the "ethical neutrality" bias has been amply documented, and needs no further discussion here. There are probably numerous initially destructive effects even in the case of like-ethnic identifications, based in latent hostilities and unconscious identification with out-group myths and prejudices. In the case of the Jewish religious affiliation, healthy and unhealthy aspects of the Jewish therapist's and patient's manifest identities may bind the two together, such as (1) self-perception as a member of a minority, (2) feelings of fear and persecution based on (1) and induced by parental upbringing, (3) warm feelings and attachment to religious rituals, (4) an obsession with being better than other members of society, and (5) sensitivity to bias. In the light of the increase of patients who are *ba'alei teshuvah* (penitents) or children of concentration camp survivors, it would be prudent for therapists who are themselves *ba'alei teshuvah* or children of camp survivors to explore the range of feelings which emerge in encountering patients of similar background. In general, the therapist's readiness to identify with and confirm his own religiosity, and to help patients do the same, would be the complementary and complicating aspect of the above aspects of identity, with significant transference and countertransference potential.

Some case illustrations will highlight the above points.

CASE 6

A 17 year-old male, religious Jewish patient was being treated by a religious therapist, both of whom belonged to the same religious community and to families with close ties. The patient had recently returned to America from Israel where he had immigrated with his family when he was 11. He had been very unhappy in Israel, got along poorly with peers and teachers, and was prone to anxiety attacks alternating with depressive periods during which times he often threatened to commit suicide. The therapist had initially consulted several times by phone with the patient's grandparents (who were in charge of his care during his stay in America) to whom he gave advice and charged no fee. Subsequently, he suggested that the patient be encouraged to seek psychotherapy, and when the patient did, the therapist was asked to elect his case.

The patient came to his initial session quite anxious and agitated, letting the therapist know that all the secular psychologists he had encountered thus far failed to appreciate the importance of religion in his life, while the religious counselors and rabbis he had encountered failed to appreciate the extent of his psychological pain. In a characteristic style, the patient demonstrated many obsessive-compulsive trends, with a defense tendency toward splitting and lapsing into deep depression. After a few sessions, the patient was able to discuss his masturbatory compulsion and disturbing sexual fantasies, but not with any adequate relinquishing of his intellectualizing or isolation.

During this period, the therapist was frequently contacted by the patient's rabbi (who was also the therapist's rabbi), the patient's teacher (who was at one time the therapist's teacher), and grandparents who all with good intentions inquired about the patient's progress. The therapist with the patient's permission gave each various amounts of confidential information, rationalizing that each was in a position to need psychological perpective on the patient. While the therapist actually had keen insight into the patient's problems, this insight was being used to obtain narcissistic gratification from the patient's and therapist's infracommunity rather than solely for the sake of the patient's well-being. The therapist had technically and factually denied the patient's individuality and need for independence at the same time that he considered these vital therapeutic goals for the patient.

Within a few sessions, the patient suddenly announced that he had decided to return to Israel. The therapist superficially questioned whether this was a healthy decision, but failed to recognize that this decision was an acting-out of negative transferential feelings evoked both by the therapist's as of yet unrecognized countertransference reactions to the patient as well as by the patient's intolerance of his increasing dependence upon the therapist. They decided to terminate therapy. Three days later, the therapist was contacted by the patient's worried grandmother who informed the therapist that the patient had decided to remain in America. The patient asked if they could resume their therapeutic contract. The therapist consented to this without at any point discussing both percipitious decisions. It was not long before the patient again decided to return to Israel, and then to change his mind again. The therapist's consistent failure to confront his own mismanagement of the patient, his anger with him, and his almost conscious relief at the thought of being free of the entangling alliance left him unable to deal with this final spate of acting-out behavior. When the patient commented that he had gained much from their work together, the therapist blandly agreed and wished him good luck.

CASE 7

An orthodox Jewish psychologist who was my supervisee took on a patient from the yeshiva (rabbinical seminary) in their community at the advice of the patient's dean, who was at one time the therapist's dean. While the therapist made meaningful initial attempts to prevent their mutual religious commitments and loyalties from contaminating therapy, significant such contamination surfaced within the first month of therapy. The therapist allowed the patient to discuss their therapeutic work with the patient's dean and, as a result, had to deal daily with the dean's anti-psychological animadversions, expressed by the patient through arguments and ruminative monologues. The therapist was spending much time engaged in philosophical debate, finding himself exhausted at the end of the hour. The therapist also found it increasingly difficult to deal with the patient's hostility and resistance and with his own resentment againt the patient and his former dean.

The therapist soon began coming late to sessions, offering the patient and his supervisor lame excuses couched in terms intended to protest his own religious commitment. For example, the therapist suddenly felt the need to rearrange his personal religious study hour to the hour just prior to his patient's session and blamed his tardiness on an inability to "tear himself away" from the exciting material he was learning. Such comments actually failed to have any appreciable "inspiring" effect upon the patient.

The therapist was unable to interpret his patient's resistance and rumination. He believed that the patient was poorly motivated and not psychologically-minded. This was only partially true. To be sure, the patient was well-defended behind intellectualizations, denials, and projections, and would no doubt remain "unmotivated" to change until such defenses were adequately dealt with. Moreover, the patient's reactions included a realistic perception of the therapist's countertransference. The patient's fantasy that he was "protected" by his mentor's surveillance from the spiritual dangers of psychotherapy was reinforced by the therapist's own fear of not being approved of and of being considered dangerous by his co-religionists.

When I confronted the therapist with these problematic behaviors, he expressed a "sense of pressure" to handle the patient with kid gloves in order "to not disfavor the profession in the eyes of the primitive yeshivah community" and his dean. This moralizing was a projection of the therapist's own superego demand for perfection and compliance, and of his own guilt over having realized through his professional career a negative self-image based on hostile attitudes toward college education he had assimilated during his own earlier years at yeshivah. He came to understand his sense of pressure as emerging from his own ambivalence toward intense religious commitment and, at the same time, from his doubts about the superiority of psychotherapy over the "inherent" curative potential of religious belief. Whereas his previous professional endeavors evoked in him a healthy sense of efficacy and satisfaction, the current religious patient (an alter ego) evoked a sense of unlove, marginality, and faithlessness. The deeper significance of the therapist's doubts lay in unresolved conflicts related to paternal authority and to intense and complicated identification with his religious dean who was in certain ways a father substitute. The curative role that the therapist had adopted as a professional identity was itself a substitute for "priestly" powers he had earlier sought through his magical identification with the dean and about which he was so intensely ambivalent.

It was not easy for the therapist to resolve his ambivalence. However, through more careful attention to his reactions with the current patient in therapy and through supervision he became less defensive about his patient's mistrust and rigidity, and he regained his independent leadership capacity in therapy. The therapist met with his former dean and informed him in a respectful manner that it was important to preserve the dyadic relationship. It took some time to win a pact of noninterference from the dean. However, when this was accomplished it effectively reduced one significant source of the patient's resistances.

In the case of the therapists discussed in the preceding vignettes, the therapists' professional and technical preferences have been surrendered in favor of personal preferences. The patient and therapist are seeking the more general and immediate rewards of monopolizing upon their unanalyzed religious familiality. Such surrender indicates mutual colusion, stimulated by the participants' religiosity and elaborated upon by intrapsychic needs and influences, to avoid exposing each other to the effortful work of exploring the deeper conflicts of the religious patient.

COUNTERTRANSFERENCE REACTIONS
TO NEWLY RELIGIOUS PATIENTS

In a recent paper, Mester and Klein (1981) discuss treatment dilemmas encountered in clinical work with young Jewish "revivalists" or newly-religious *ba'alei teshuvah*. The authors successfully demonstrate how patients' religious beliefs effect the therapeutic atmosphere. In particular, Mester and Klein emphasize that therapists' countertransference reactions need to be carefully restrained so as to minimize their potentially destructive influence on the course and quality of psychotherapy. I have tried to emphasize that countertransference reactions eventually can serve in a constructive and diagnostic capacity, so long as the therapist appropriately calibrates and differentiates his reactions from contaminating influences such as personal attitudes and views about religion and, more importantly, from the dynamic factors in therapists' own personalities which are addressed to one degree or another by religious belief and its qualities and intensities (e.g., transitional qualities, themes of power, etc.). In this regard, the narcissistic, aggressive, iconoclastic and fanatically dogmatic tendencies common among newly-religious personalities require special attention.

Mester and Klein articulate several distinct countertransference reactions. Two that merit additional comment are the therapist's feeling of being passively manipulated by the patient into the position of persecutor/punisher and feeling "envious" of the patient's new-found religious sense of belonging and direction. Regarding the feeling of being manipulated, the therapist must reflect on the possibility that others in the newly-religious devotee's interpersonal community are likewise manipulated or driven to feel this way as a result of the patient's unconscious effort to relinquish choice and responsibility, to extract narcissistic supplies, or to test out potentially idealizeable objects with whom to replace objects whose love the patient may be losing, or whom he entirely loses, or with whom identification is painful. In still other instances, this unconscious technique on the patient's part is designed to project anxiety-provoking qualities which emerge as the devotee aggressively rejects former ties (or self-images) or abandons former personality traits no longer compatible with his currently adopted "religious" self-image or identifications. This latter dynamic is quite important. I often have found it a clue to the patient's failure to successfully mourn these abondoned qualities, loyalties, or representations as he attempts instead merely to "dump" them, as if this could occur without also losing some valued part of self structure. Finally, for many Jewish penitents, the role of *ba'al teshuvah* is often cathected as some kind of "badge of courage" which for many seems to include the belief—partly reinforced by popular stereotype—that they are a lonely and persecuted group. This dynamic role often has sadistic and masochistic motives. This image is self-fulfillingly reinforced by unconsciously or consciously provoking others' unease, anger, impatience, and withdrawal.

Regarding the countertransference reaction of "envy," Mester and Klein relate the clinician's feelings to the "unconscious and/or preconscious conviction that the patients had reached the ultimate psychological solution to existential doubting and emotional pains" (1981, p. 300). I have invariably found such radical solving of doubt either to be only apparent—thinly masking a plague of doubt beneath the veneer of confidence and self-assurredness—or attributeable to outright and heavy-handed denial. Hidden under many so-called existential doubts lie exquisite psychological doubts, shame, insecurity, and anomie. When this is the case, a religious devotee's "enviable" sense of conviction may be, at least initially, a reaction-formation or inversion of some kind (see Case 5). Since further problems lie ahead for the religious penitent who merely suppresses doubt and anxiety—especially the doubts and anxieties which motivated the initial religious development—therapists must carefully explore rather than take for granted such countertransference reactions.

MANAGEMENT OF COUNTERTRANSFERENCE WITH THE RELIGIOUS PATIENT

The following practice techniques should help reduce the distortive effects of dissimilar or like-religious affiliation among therapists and patients:

1. The therapist must develop a consistent conceptual understanding of both neurotic and normal needs for religion, including an understanding of the potential conflict-bearing nature of his religion's attitudes toward other-worldliness and this-worldliness, attitudes about God, ethics, the effects of religious belief in coping with problems surrounding death and loss, superego aspects *versus* narcissistic qualities, and so forth.

2. The therapist must be able to differentiate autonomous religious belief from dysautonomous belief and the way in which legitimate beliefs and practices are used as resistances. This will enable him to appreciate when his own beliefs and practices motivate either over-interest or refusal to deal with certain material which emerges during therapy.

3. In addition, the therapist must be willing and able to tolerate the patient's normal need for an area of emotional and not necessarily rational commitment and contain his need to impart "insight" into every aspect of the patient's religious life.

4. The therapist must be willing to analyze his own beliefs in terms of the above three factors.

5. The therapist should develop a nonanxious and benevolent attitude about his own anger, anxiety, and frustration when encountering religious patients with pathologic or merely "strange" beliefs.

6. The therapist must clarify at the outset of therapy that the beliefs, values, and practices shared by himself and the patient are as much subject to positive and negative feelings as any other aspect of their lives, and that these will rightfully be subjected to their mutual scrutiny.

As these ground rules are presented to the religious patient, the therapist should monitor the quality of his own reactions and associations to the patient's responses to these early expectations. He should check for tendencies on his part to fill gaps in his understanding of the patient's behavior with presumptions about religious personalities in general, as well as subtle tendencies to disregard religious mannerisms which he believes are nonrelevant to therapeutic work, or are "sufficiently understood."

When countertransference reactions are recognized during

therapy, these are best managed in three steps: (1) The therapist must modify the underlying basis in himself for the difficulty, (2) correct the effects of the error or mismanagement in the session, and (3) determine and explore the patient's response to the therapist's error (see Langs, 1982).

CASE 6 (CONTINUED)

The destructive countertransference reaction in the case of the 17 year-old male actually resulted in both parties bolting from their misalliance. The patient did, however, attempt once again to establish a therapeutic alliance. By this time, the therapist had become more experienced with his feelings and more aware of the negative influence of his own reactions. He had achieved a *modus operandi* whereby he was able to limit his need for narcissistic gratification through his professional involvement within his own community. This involved a considerable amount of self-growth. In their new initial session, the therapist raised the issue of his discussions with the patient's grandparents and teacher, and allowed the patient to express his resentment toward all concerned. Accepting the patient's anger and validity of his need for confidentiality, the therapist explored the destabilizing effect of the patient's earlier decisions about Israel. He carefully raised the possibility that these decisions were reactions to the therapist's apparent disinterest in the integrity of their relationship. The patient was able to acknowledge this and began to recall his associations at the time of these percipitous decisions. The therapist was then able to use this work as an example of the value of expressing feelings verbally rather than acting them out.

PSYCHOLOGICAL TESTING

The emergence of religious symbols, idioms, and ideas during the process of psychological testing also raises several important clinical concerns. Experience indicates that one can expect some religious expressions unique to the patient's lifestyle to emerge during testing, whose diagnostic meaning depends on several factors (Draper, et al, 1965).

The most frequent and least diagnostically significant religious expressions are the everyday terminology and forms of linguistic expression that are an autonomous characteristic of the patient's parlance. These would be encountered in regular conversation with such persons, during their dialogue during treatment, and during testing. In the case of orthodox Jewish patients, examples include liberal sprinklings of Yiddish expressions which have become part of their manner of speech and are occasionally used as substitutes for English expression even among persons who speak English quite well. This will be more pronounced among persons with yeshivah background and persons living in religious communities which continue to be strongly influenced by Eastern European Jewish habits and customs.

However, within the subset of idioms and other such characteristics that can be considered normative for the particular group of religious persons being tested, there are departures from such norms which may have clinical significance. In establishing the importance of these departures, the clinician must have broad familiarity with the subgroup's normative behavior in order to be able accurately to differentiate departures which would be acceptable within the subgroup, and which may not alter the meaning of tests on which such persons produced these sorts of responses, from other departures, normative within the subgroup, which do in fact call for alternative interpretations of tests, and departures which would be deemed abnormal even within the subgroup's perspective. The search for subgroup norms on standard psychodiagnostic instruments has an important function, but cannot fully supplant the important and useful qualitative perspectives gained by comparison of the individual subculture member's test responses against national or multi-nationally-derived norms or the need to report the findings of such comparisons (Anastasi, 1976; Munday & Rosenberg, 1979; Sundberg & Gonzales, 1981). How such departures are reported and interpreted will largely depend on such factors as: (a) Are the tests being utilized for the purpose of gauging abilities relative to the needs of some institution which operates within national norms (e.g., the

American school system) or one which operates primarily within subgroup norms (e.g., a private religious school where certain academic subjects are less emphasized, or are emphasized at a slower pace than Hebrew subjects)? (b) Is one utilizing tests of fairly universal abilities or which are based on certain assumptions about universal qualities of normal ego functioning (e.g., the Rorschach) where subgroup members' departures from "normal" behavior may indeed retain their full clinical import despite some subtle uniquenesses in content or style? These questions in and of themselves may not directly point to the correct attitude for the examiner if he or she does not also have a good deal of experience with the particular subgroup.

The diagnostic relevance of the preceding discussion was actually anticipated by Rapaport, Gill, and Schafer, illustrated in their discussion of the diagnostic significance of Picture-Completion subtest of the Wechsler-Bellvue (1968, p. 133):

> How a query for information replaces concentration and defeats the subject is clearly illustrated in an obsessional patient of orthodox Jewish rearing who on no. 6 (a picture of a pig missing a tail) asked, "Do pigs have tails?" Apparently he had discovered that the missing element was the tail; but instead of relying on the results of his scrutiny, as a good obsessive doubter he wanted the approval of authority — which probably due to his rearing he did not have.

In other words, since it is doubtful that the subject in this example truly lacked knowledge of such generally available information, his obsessive style becomes even more apparent, as it evidently did on other test items as well. Diagnostically, the subject's doubt cannot be excused merely as veritable lack of knowledge, and this is so despite the possibility of cultural influence. I might add, tangential to this particular example, that among *young* children from very orthodox Jewish homes, it is common that even nine or ten year-old subjects in fact do not know "from what animal do we get bacon?" [WISC-R, Information No. 9]. Of course, the failure of this item alone will not significantly alter such an individual's Verbal Subscale IQ or Full Scale IQ score, or the import of the score. It is quite another matter, however, when the child does seem to have this information, but appears embarrassed to produce such knowledge, or adds derogatory comments, and so forth, as will be illustrated below.

I have explored and illustrated these issues in great detail elsewhere and will provide here one rich clinical example which I think illustrates the type of attention one needs to give to the emergence of idiographic religious expression during testing (Spero, 1984). Following the clinical material, I will offer some diagnostic principles which I believe aid in the development of appropriate sensitivity to subgroup behavior during testing and in the proper interpretation of such behaviors.

CASE 8

Devoutly orthodox religious patients may react contentiously to the need for psychological testing by questioning such tests' validity or applicability to them, "given" their religious uniqueness, or by questioning the religious integrity of the examiner. Generally, contentious reactions will be sprinkled with allusions to deeper doubts or disrespect for psychology as a science and profession. Sometimes these reactions are expressed only after testing has begun and upon experiencing some unease with a particular test. In the case of religious Jewish patients, such reactions typically are ensconced in terms of the subjects' interpretations of Jewish morals and beliefs. When this occurs, the clinical approach becomes complicated, because it is not initially clear whether these reactions in fact are valid arguments designed to protect authentic moral sensitivities or pseudo-religious ones which mask neurotic disturbances. Furthermore, when an examinee directly questions the examiner's moral and religious scruples—and if inappropriately understood and managed—the examiner may experience a host of negative countertransferential feelings which may cloud his clinical perceptions and disable him from working effectively with the particular patient (see Pruyser, 1976; Walker & Firetto, 1965).

The subject to be discussed is a 23 year-old male who since high school has been a student in an intensely orthodox yeshivah in Israel. He attended this institution for four years prior to referral.

The patient left Israel ostensibly due to a clash with fellow students whom he felt did not respect his privacy or his unique religious perspectives. While the subject's parents maintain a kosher home and are moderately observant of Shabbat, the young man described himself as more *frum* (observant) and knowledgeable than they.

Upon returning home from Israel, the patient described himself as "perhaps a bit depressed and indecisive," but also adamant about not going to college. He wanted very much to return to yeshivah studies. In filling in other details about the "episode" in Israel, the subject appeared to have experienced a manic reaction. His parents described that the patient had recently begun grimmacing in a strange way, and that the young man's father's brother was an institutionalized schizophrenic.

I administered first the *Bender-Gestalt* which went without major difficulty and revealed no sign of organic disturbance. However, I noted one serious rotation and also that the subject experienced difficulty when copying the elongated, crossed, sharp-edged design (item no. 7) making numerous erasures and redrawings, which is sometimes suggestive of anxiety concerning sexual stimuli. The *Minnesota Percepto-Diagnostic Test* was then administered, again with no major difficulties, although the same difficulty with sharp-edged designs were observed, and the overall score lay in the neurotic disturbance range.

I then administered the Draw-a-Person task. The subject first drew a figure identified as a male. The "male" had no facial features, and even following my testing-of-the-limits, the subject felt his rendering needed no modification. I then instructed him to draw a female. The subject hesitated and became visibly upset. After 40 seconds of blank staring at the paper, the subject looked at me very seriously and exclaimed, "To tell you the truth, this is very odd...I mean, why do I have to draw a woman? It's disgusting, to say the least! You know, at first I didn't mind, but what do these tests have to do with me? These are tests that you probably got from your college background which have nothing to do with the *neshameh* [soul] of a Jewish person." The subject further questioned what could possibly be learned by having him draw a woman, and did I feel that this request was *tzniusdik* (modest)? I responded merely by saying that I needed to sample different aspects of his life, and that in order for me to do my job, it would be important that he try to follow my instructions as best he could.

The subject hesitated for a few seconds, acknowledged that he was no artist, and proceeded to draw a female on the same sheet of paper. The picture he drew essentially was identical to the male figure, with long hair and an outline of a dress alongside the body. He did not attempt to erase the "male" figure beneath the dress. However, the female figure was drawn with some facial features. When next asked to draw a picture of himself, the young man responded that the first figure was himself. In describing the "persons" he had drawn, the subject remarked that the male "lacked character" which he explained only by comparison to the female who had "more personal strength...as you can see from her face." The subject still made no changes on the first drawing. And again, on the Draw-a-Family task, he drew two males with no facial features, while the females had facial features. There was now the stronger suggestion of inadequate sexual differentiation, the possibility of depersonalization, and a disturbed quality of object representations. The concrete way the subject described the figures' character also bore the grim spectre of schizophrenic process.

During the WAIS-R information subtest, the patient responded as follows to item no. 18 ("What is the main theme of the book of Genesis?"): "Well...it tells the story of creation through the development of the Jewish people." This response is correct, and the inclusion of specific reference to Jewish people is appropriate in the present context. Further, there was no other indication of a tendency to overinclude or overelaborate in the subject's responses throughout the remainder of the test, which gives additional reason to be unconcerned about this specific response.

On the Picture Arrangement subtest, the subject completed the tasks in a tedious but correct fashion, until the cards for item no. 7 were laid out before him (this item, new in the WAIS-R, depicts a man helping two women in succession up a small hill). The patient fumbled with the cards, put them in their correct sequence, and then sat back. He once again began an onslaught against the examiner, referring pointedly to his obligation to be examined by a pious Jew. At this point, I wondered aloud whether the subject felt he had been incorrectly advised about seeing me in particular. This he denied, but railed now against the validity of "tests made for *goyim* [non-Jews] and for people whose minds are more attuned to the stuff on these cards! If you want to know about my feelings and *hashakafot* [religious perspectives], ask me and I'll tell you. I can tell you right now that I won't come if this is the stuff we're going to discuss. Dr. _____ in Israel would never give such tests to a yeshivah student. Even the *goyisheh* psychiatrist in [his home town] that I went to once didn't bother with such tests! I resent the whole thing!"

I tried through analogies (e.g., do Jews require separate driving tests?) and in other ways to make it clear to the subject that the tests were merely a baseline of skills common to all persons, and were not intended to tap his spiritual beliefs or alter them in any way. I assured him that he would have ample opportunity to share these with me in a direct fashion — and at that time the differences between himself and non-Jewish persons could be emphasized if he so desired. The subject seemed to collect himself, but then added that, "If the [rabbinic luminary] knew I was taking these tests, he would yank me right outa here!" To this I remarked that I would be more than happy to explain my tests and their rationale to this rabbinic authority so that he could perhaps better advise the subject whether he could indeed participate in these specific tests. Surprisingly, the young man responded, "No. Let's just get on with the testing."

I will conclude this detailed case illustration with some material drawn from the subject's Rorschach protocol. (The location scores included in the verbatim quotations follow Klopfer's system.) On Card III, the subject broke the gestalt into several large detail responses: "[35"] This reminds me of *Mishnat ha-Mapelet* in *Masekhet Niddah* [the chapter in talmudic tractate *Niddah* which deals with miscarriages from the standpoint of the laws of family purity]...[12"]. Here [D5] is a *nefel* [a dead child or fetus], you know, a child that, *rahmanah litzlan* [Heaven forfend!], uh...here [tiny, lighter shaded area in upper third of D5] is its eye. This [D3] is the *shilyah* [placenta] that came out with it...This [D6], is, uh, these two are dead, I don't know, *ke'min oaf* [an abortus that has the appearance of a chick]. That's all...Oh, to, uh, do something with these [D2], this is blood, the *hatikhat dam* [clum of blood]." This treatment suggest color shock, both in the way the blot is broken into details and in the way color and shading are dealt with. "Blood" verbalizations, confabulation, and fabulized imputations of symbolic forces at work also occurred in other of the subject's responses. Thus, from the clinical standpoint, the erudite talmudic references must be deemed gratuitous and little modify the standard inferences that must be drawn from such a response on a card where most people see whole human figures. The subject's organizing processes are disturbed and have merely utilized familiar idioms and symbols in the rapidly deteriorating attempt to deal with the impact of this particular blot.

Several points are illustrated in the preceding case selection. First, I would emphasize as far as concerns the technique of managing patient's "religious" resistances during testing that I attempt merely to gain the individual's compliance rather than to fully explore with the patient the meaning of such resistances as I would do during psychotherapy. I also am not adverse to the use of directive approaches to secure compliance with testing, such as offering the patient my interpretation of the acceptability of psychological testing according to Jewish ethics or to recommend that the issue be discussed with his or her religious advisors, whereas I am particularly opposed to this approach during treatment. At the same time, when a direct approach is not greeted with quick compliance, it is important that further remonstration not occur which is likely to result in negative feelings on the part of both participants. Should a patient continue to refuse to engage in the testing process, this should be communicated to the referral source and, if possible, different arrangements made. Fortunately, extreme resistance is rare.

A second point concerns the nature of the subject's apparently religious or ethical justifications for criticizing or refusing to participate in testing. One recalls the mythic patient who objected to psychological tests on the grounds that the examiner was upsetting him with "those dirty cards." The understanding has always been, based on the projective hypothesis, that such reactions are a product of the subject's inner conflicts and not the result of "dirty" stimuli. The religious perspective also subscribes to the idea that the range of stimuli represented by the real world does not necessarily evoke indigenously negative or "dirty" responses, although some individuals may indeed make such responses. To use a simple but useful example, Jewish law has never objected to appropriately conducted gynecological examinations and would regard as unwarranted and abnormal an extremely vociferous objection to such examinations, even if couched in terms of Judaism's laws of modesty. I believe the same rationale applies to psychological testing, which means that undue resistance to working with the standard tests currently used could readily be viewed with an eye toward some kind of difficulty on the patient's part.

A third consideration bears on the clinical interpretation of the religious material which emerges during the testing process, such as emerged in the case of the patient under discussion. For example, while it would not be surprising if a Jew raised in ultra-orthodox circles referred to non-Jews as *goyim* (which translates as "nations"), it is noteworthy how this patient uses the term in an emotionally charged way to disown devalued aspects of self and to disqualify the applicability of the tests to himself. In the patient's response to Rorschach card III, the references to the abortus do indeed come from essentially legalistic knowledge acquired during rabbinical training. However, one would argue that card III does not necessarily look like an abortus and so forth anymore than it necessarily looks like "two women standing over a brazier," the more or less typical response. A universal principle is in operation when an individual from any religious persuasion attempts to make sense of the inkblot, and that is that his ego will bring to bear whatever inner experiences and preferred methods of perceiving and organizing ambiguity are available to him. Typically, one organizes the world in a way that is pleasant, consensual, and easy for others to empathize with. In a sense, with such a patient one must wonder why he was not able to deal with the impact of card III by calling forth the wealth of additional symbols and topics that are scattered throughout the Talmud or in his own life. Like the physician-subject, this rabbinical student as a result of his specialization understandably has greater familiarity than other persons with the grim details of miscarriages and so forth. However, the clinical focus is drawn to his apparent preference for such details and to his particularly inadequate use of such details in making sense of the blot compared to the norm. I believe this perspective must be applied to the emergence of religious material throughout the testing and treatment process.

The following guidelines are useful for understanding the meaning of religious material which emerges during testing.

(1) The examiner must have thorough familiarity with the idiom, mannerisms, law, and lore of the religious subgroups he examines, as well as a complete understanding of the purposes and implications of normative responses for the instruments he utilizes in order to better appreciate when a non-normative response is essentially the same as that which he is seeking and when it is not. Even when a non-normative response is deemed essentially adequate, such responses, and certainly a preference for such responses, merit note and report.

(2) Attention should be given to qualitative aspects of the emergence of religious material, including content, accompanying feeling states, and the examinee's expressed attitude toward such religious content (e.g., praising, derogatory, belittling). These nuances always shed a great deal of light upon the quality of the examinee's use of and identification with religious material.

(3) Clinicians are accustomed to inferring from the patient's material the quality of object relationships, potential modes of transference, and other intra- and interpersonal dynamics which exist and may be expected during treatment. This kind of inference drawing is no less important with religious patients, but should be broadened in scope whenever possible to include all possible inference about the nature and quality of the patient's attitude and relationship with religious authorities and divinity figures.

(4) When religious material includes moralizing and the expression of symbolization, care should be given to the quality, form, and amount. Given that the spontaneous production of symbolic responses on certain tests, such as the Rorschach, has potentially pathognomic significance, the examiner must differentiate between appropriate expression and that which

has become a substitute for constructive reality testing.

SUMMARY

Several diagnostic guidelines have been offered in order to enhance the recognition of dysautonomous religious practice and belief and the ability to discriminate such religiosity from mature religiosity which may contain but typically transcends its infantile underpinnings. These guidelines also will help to differentiate healthy religiosity from less healthy psychological undercurrents. Practice principles for diagnostic testing and treatment have been suggested, which include several procedures for lessening the potentially distortive influence of the patient's and the therapist's religious attitudes and feelings.

REFERENCES

Anastasi, A. *Psychological Testing.* New York: Macmillan, 1976.

Draper, E., Meyer, G., Prazen, Z. & Samuelson, G. On the diagnostic value of religious ideation. *Archives of General Psychiatry*, 1965, *13*, 202-207.

Guntrip, H. *Schizoid Phenomenon, Object Relations, and the Self.* New York: International Universities Press, 1969.

Krasner, B. Religious loyalties in clinical work: A contextual view. *Journal of Jewish Communal Service*, 1981-82, *58*, 108-115.

Langs, R. *Psychotherapy.* New York: Aronson, 1982.

Mester, R. & Klein, H. The young Jewish revivalist: A therapist's dilemma. *British Journal of Medical Psychology*, 1981, *54*, 299-306.

Munday, L. & Rosenberg, G. *Social Concerns and the Stanford-Binet.* Illinois: Riverside Publishing Co., 1979.

Pruyser, P. *The Minister As Diagnotician.* Phila.: Westminster, 1976.

Pruyser, P. The seamy side of current religious belief. *Bulletin of the Menninger Clinic*, 1977, *41*, 329-340.

Rapaport, D., Gill., M. & Schafer, R. *Diagnostic Psychological Testing.* New York: International Universities Press, 1968.

Rizzuto, A.M. *The Birth of the Living God: A Psychoanalytic Study.* Chicago: University of Chicago Press, 1979.

Sevensky, R. Religion, psychology, and mental health. *American Journal of Psy-*

    chotherapy, 1984, *38*, 73-86.
Spero, M.H. The clinical significance of orthodox Jewish cultural content in idio-
    graphic responses to diagnostic psychological tests. *Journal of Psychology and Ju-
    daism*, 1984, *8*, in press.
Spero, M.H. The contemporary penitent personality: Diagnostic, treatment,
    and some ethical considerations. *Journal of Psychology and Judaism*, 1980, *4*,
    133-193.
Spero, M.H. Individual psychotherapeutic treatment of the cult personality. In
    D. Halperin (ed.), *Psychodynamic Perspectives on Religion, Sect, and Cult*. Little-
    ton, Mass.: John Wright/PSG Publishing Co., 1983.
Sundberg, N. & Gonzales, L. Cross-cultural and cross-ethnic assessment. In R.
    McReynolds (ed.), *Advances in Psychological Assessment. Vol. 5*. San Francisco:
    Jossey-Bass, 1981.
Walker, R.E. & Firetto, A. The clergyman as a variable in psychological testing.
    Journal for the Scientific Study of Religion, 1965, *4*, 234-239.

Section Three
TRANSFERENCE, COUNTERTRANS-
FERENCE, AND THE ALLIANCE

Chapter 3

CLINICAL INTERSECTIONS BETWEEN THE RELIGION OF THE PSYCHIATRIST AND HIS PATIENTS

JOHN R. PETEET, M.D.

A GROWING literature addresses the relationship between religion and psychology, from a variety of points of view (James, 1902; Freud, 1928; Allport, 1950; Rizutto, 1974; Reiff, 1959). Recently, increased clinical attention to psychotherapy of religious patients has included discussion of the role of religion in patients' lives (Pruyser, 1971; Spero, 1976; Levin and Zegans, 1974; Cohen and Smith, 1976), the social role of the psychotherapist (London, 1976; Halleck, 1976; Pattison, 1966), and countertransference and other issues which arise in the treatment of such persons (Apolito, 1970; McLemore and Court, 1977: Peteet, 1981; Spero, 1981). This chapter discusses in detail some of the decisions faced by the religious psychotherapists of religious patients. Most of the examples are drawn from my practice as a Christian psychiatrist in a major urban area where I am regularly referred patients who want to see a therapist of the same faith.

INITIAL TREATMENT CONSIDERATIONS

One of the first decisions a therapist faces is whether to accept a patient in treatment or to refer the patient elsewhere. Several factors play a part in this decision. One is the match between a patient's clinical need and the therapist's ability to meet it. For example (Case 1), a 25 year-old, single, white male working in a fast-food restaurant came to me for an evaluation and help with his violent fantasies toward women. He also was afraid of acting out these impulses, which began several years earlier following an incident of rejection by a woman. He stated he was looking for a Christian psychiatrist because he wanted someone who understood both his desperation and his recent conversion to Christianity.

He began to describe a deprived early childhood, a history of having dropped out of high school, abusing a number of drugs, working odd jobs, and living with a homosexual alcoholic. Several months prior to therapy, he was taken in by a Pentocostal church and was "born again." When the church's prayers for healing of his distress were not answered to his satisfaction, the church referred him indirectly to me. In his initial interview, the patient questioned whether I knew his pastor and wondered whether I was "born again." He then went on to express considerable ambivalence toward the church. On one hand, he was fearful of losing its support and the promise of forgiveness ("because God won't accept anyone who isn't righteous"); on the other hand, he was afraid of being unable to live up to its strict standards of behavior (e.g., no sex before marriage). Several months prior to calling me, he had been seen for three months at a local state mental health center by a psychiatric resident who subsequently left and then by a psychopharmacologist at another hospital to whom he owed several hundred dollars. He also had been admitted for one day to a state hospital after having expressed fears of losing control, though there was neither evidence that he had been actively psychotic nor that he benefitted from medication.

In reviewing this history with the patient, I discussed with him the emotional and financial difficulties he had incurred in his previous attempts to sustain private psychotherapy and agreed to see him in clinic on a weekly basis. I also agreed initially that it could be helpful for him to see a therapist who appreciated his religious struggles. However, the patient soon began to miss appointments and then called, wanting to be seen and to be admitted to the hospital for a "rest." With his borderline character difficulties and his crisis of confidence in the church's ability to support him, it became apparent that more than he needed a Christian psychiatrist, he simply needed a person he could afford to see consistently who also was part of an institution which could evaluate him in an emergency and provide hospitalization or other support. Accordingly, I referred the patient to the local mental health center where he had been followed before and offered to consult with his treatment team if specific religious issues arose which required a Christian perspective.

A related consideration in deciding whether a religious therapist indeed offers religious patients a significant advantage over another therapist is the patient's ability to trust a non-religious therapist. Sometimes, the patient's prior experience with therapists or religious counselors provides important background in making this assessment.

As an example (Case 2), a 21 year-old conservative Christian college junior with a history of a previous psychotic episode and hospitalization was reluctant to see a psychiatrist because he had been told during his hospitalization that he was "too religious." Indeed, the discharge summary from that hospital admission confirmed that "the treatment plan focused on a reduction of his religious preoccupation." The patient eventually agreed to see a Christian psychiatrist and was referred to this author by his pastor. A year later, after graduating from college and now unsure whether to enter the ministry or business, the patient experienced another brief psychotic episode. He subsequently moved to his home in a neighboring state, at which point he saw a non-religious psychiatrist primarily for medication. However, because of the favorable alliance which he had established earlier with this author, he found it worthwhile to return from out-of-state to see him every few weeks. During the period of this new work, the patient was able to assume more responsibility in the family business and became seriously involved with a woman. Although this arrangement was somewhat unwieldy at times, it proved to be stable over a period of years.

It was apparently important for the above patient to feel he had a special relationship with a therapist by virtue of their shared religious experience and faith. However, the same need can make certain kinds of therapeutic work impractical. For example, a patient may choose a therapist he feels he can trust because of pre-existing and ongoing religious and social contact with that professional. Consider in this regard a 30 year-old, married, temporarily employed librarian (Case 3) who attended the same church as her future therapist. The relationship was close enough that she had invited him to her wedding. When she elected therapy with this professional, her presenting problems were "overwhelming feelings of anxiety and guilt" due to an experience in her current life which revived earlier experiences of parental deprivation and misunderstanding. She felt relieved to be able to confide in a therapist she knew, whom she felt could understand the importance of her faith in her career struggles (she had spent two years in the lay ministry) and in her marriage (she had met her husband through shared church work), and would not criticize her for this as had her family (which viewed her as an unrealistic religious fanatic). However, she soon felt awkward about discussing her disagreements with her husband, in particular their sexual difficulties. The therapist discussed the tension between their dual roles and encouraged her referral to a colleague while offering to remain in touch with the patient and her new therapist to be certain she was satisfied. Fortunately, he was able to find a colleague with a similar religious background and an interest in the treatment of religious patients, and the patient was able to make the transition without feeling undue rejection.

A third consideration in electing to treat the religious patient is the patient's need for integrating psychological and religious aspects of himself and the therapist's ability to meet that need. A 30 year-old, unmarried seminary professor (Case 4) referred by her internist for depression, provides an example. This patient was a reserved, perfectionistic person raised in a missionary home who felt the call to an academic, religious vocation. She enjoyed research much more than teaching and became frustrated and depressed, with thoughts of suicide, when the only available job she could find was a demanding teaching position located far from friends and family. Yet, she regarded doing her best as a duty to God and viewed ways of relieving her sense of pressure as legitimate only if she had a fully disabling medical problem. As she bagan to feel desperate and unable to concentrate on her work, she sought out an endocrinologist. When he raised the possibility of psychiatric consultation, she objected on the grounds that previous therapists whom she had been asked to see for similar difficulties had been unsympathetic to the religious imperatives she felt and that she would only be able to discuss her most important conflicts with someone who shared a belief in the primary importance of one's duty to God. Her physician referred her to a Christian therapist who she was relieved to find both respected her beliefs and happened to have a personal familiarity with several aspects of her background, such as the location where she had grown up, the university she had attended, and the distinctiveness of her denomination's theology which she was attempting to preserve through her academic research.

The therapist's personal interest in integrating his sense of responsibility to God with an allowance for his human limitations made him particularly able to empathize with the patient's struggle and to indicate that he understood and respected her struggle. Conversely, the patient's integrity served as an inspiration for him and lent another perspective to his own attempts at integration. Since the patient expected herself to be able to handle life's demands without reliance on professionals, unless her abililty to work was severely threatened, she asked if she could call when she needed an appointment rather than to schedule them on a regular basis. The therapist thought this a reasonable plan, so long as she called before she felt completely desperate. He also encouraged her to find some time for herself and with friends, so she could better maintain her involvement in her work — hopefully as a challenge and not merely as a burden. While her idealistic religious beliefs, her perfectionistic personality, and her previous negative experiences with therapy all made regular psychotherapy problematic, the therapist's express appreciation for all these factors allowed him to work with her in a way which promoted rather than impaired her integration as a person.

Once engaged in treatment, a shared religious faith can have important effects on both therapist and patient. Potential advantages for the patient include an additional level of respect, trust, shared values, understanding, and the potential for the therapist to serve as a model for integration. Advantages for the therapist include the opportunity to learn from the experience of treating patients with a variety of religious beliefs and sensitivities and even from treating others with religious conflicts similar to his own and to feel he is making a unique contribution to their care.

For example (Case 5), a 35 year-old architect and father of three came for treatment to better understand his sexual identity. His wife had left him several months prior to therapy after many years of conflict concerning his homosexual behavior. Raised a nominal Catholic, the patient met his wife during the days of campus unrest in the late 1960s during which time they both rebelled against "establishment" values, living in campgrounds and informal communes. The patient later bacame more religious through the preaching of a well-known Protestant evangelist but attended church irregularly. At the time he came for therapy, he felt a sense of personal relatedness to God as an at times sympathetic, perhaps indulgent, but at other times judgmental figure. This was reflected in his ambivalent attitude toward his homosexual behavior. He would say, "I know it's bad behavior God would condemn, so I try not to let myself be tempted by the thought," then would admit to having acted upon homosexual impulses because "it felt right at the time," and "like I would be denying a real part of myself not to," which he felt God also would not want. He first investigated treatment at a gay counseling center but felt his moral and religious struggles were not being addressed there and so found this author as a Christian therapist who he hoped would help him reconcile his conflict.

The therapist was initially somewhat tempted to respond with his own view on the theology of homosexuality but was curbed by a stronger awareness of the patient's need to speak with someone who would not impose expectations. On the other hand, the therapist's attempts to help the patient understand his behavior in psychological terms were hindered by the patient's tendency to see the issues wholly in moral and religious terms. As a result, the therapist focused on two major related issues: the patient's basis for believing his homosexual behavior was unacceptable to God, and his tendency to react to others' expectations (his mother's, his wife's, his church's, or his therapist's) and to impulsively pursue brief homosexual encounters as an escape from the pressure exerted by these expectations.

At the same time, the therapist encouraged the patient to think through and develop confidence in his own choices—in particular, whether or not to pursue a homosexual life style. As a way of helping him to consider various options within the framework of the Christian faith, yet without endorsing any one choice for the patient, the therapist provided him with a Christian periodical devoted to the personal struggles of Christian homosexuals who reached different resolutions. The patient continued to occasionally express rueful frustration that the therapist could not simply tell him the right answer but found intriguing the range of perspectives in the periodical, and he began to evaluate his sexual behavior in terms of the quality of relationships it fostered. At the end of a year-long treatment, he expressed appreciation for the therapist's acceptance of both his personal limitations and his need to be true to his faith, which had allowed him to think more clearly about the values inherent in his sexual choices and to feel for the first time that these decisions were his to make. His regard both for the therapist as a psychological expert and as a Christian appeared to be a major factor in this process. The process was gratifying for the therapist because of his particularcontribution to the patient's progress and because it afforded him the opportunity to consider more deeply and concretely the religious and moral dilemmas of persons struggling with such sexual choices.

TRANSFERENCE CONSIDERATIONS

Strongly positive, negative, or ambivalent transference responses which are stimulated in part by the therapist's identity as a religious person can be problematic for both patient and therapist. Ambivalence can be considerable toward the religious therapist who comes to represent a religious or other authority figure. For example (Case 6), a 30 year-old engineer was referred by his internist for depression which had become more severe since his parents' divorce and a break-up with a girlfriend two years before. He was the only son of a fundamentalist minister whom the patient described as rigid, distant, and physically abusive to him and his sister, never apologizing but self-righteously justifying his behavior in religious terms. After obtaining a master's degree in engineering, the patient became an unordained minister for a year in his father's denomination, then returned to engineering and to an only peripheral relationship with the church.

The patient sought out a religious therapist who he hoped would understand his religious past. However, as the therapy progressed, the patient showed considerable ambivalence toward the therapist and toward both his own and the therapist's religious identification. At times, he expressed a wish to jog or play tennis with the therapist and to know more about how the therapist dealt with certain personal and theological dilemmas. At other times, when the therapist asked for the patient's thoughts about questions he had posed to the therapist (such as why he was more depressed at a particular time or whether the religious teachings he had received about God's judgment were believable), the patient half-jokingly, but sarcastically, referred to the therapist as a withholding, manipulative "shrink" with an easy job. The therapist's formulation was that the patient had been so traumatized by previous authority figures that he needed to experience the therapist as a "real person" in order to trust him. Thus, the therapist attempted to be open with his own thoughts and feelings when asked and to gently approach painful issues.

Initially, this approach seemed successful. The patient recovered from his depression and became more regular in his eating, work, and exercise habits, partly through an acknowledged identification with the therapist who the patient observed was fit, jogged, and successful in his work. The patient then made his chronic insomnia a major focus of discussion. The therapist referred him to a sleep specialist whom the patient saw with good results over a period of a few months and with whom he discussed his ambivalent feelings of admiration and competitive rivalry toward the therapist. He then returned to treatment on a monthly basis, discussing primarily his relationship with a girlfriend, which was not progressing, and his considerable success at gambling, which was unacceptable to both her family and his ideal view of himself. After finally deciding to give up both the girlfriend and gambling, he came less often for appointments.

He began one particular session by asking the therapist to indicate what his major problems were, partly to see if the therapist "had really been listening." The therapist briefly reviewed the several areas in which the patient had made progress (which included his depression, insomnia, intermittent drug abuse, overweight, relationships with women, self-discipline problems, and the roots of these problems in his childhood experience). However, the patient insisted that the therapist declare himself regarding the "major" issue remaining to be resolved, hinting that he had not yet talked much about it. The therapist felt it prudent at this point to "perform" or risk being devalued by the patient as unable to "read" him and ventured the guess that religious issues were still very troubling to the patient. He responded by questioning the therapist about his own religious beliefs (Could he really believe in a God who allowed the Holocaust? If one took a less than literal view of Jesus' statements, was not one manipulating them to suit one's own purposes?). On the defensive but hoping that the patient would soften as he had done before with a demonstration of openness, the therapist attempted to carefully share a brief rationale for his beliefs. However, the patient seemed to take this as only a confirmation of their religious differences and left without definite plans for another visit. In a belated parting postcard from a vacation place in Europe, he indicated that he had found another therapist, would like to see his former therapist on a friendly basis at the therapist's convenience, and that he appreciated his help even though he had found him cold at times.

In retrospect, the therapist in this case had underestimated the influence of the patient's anger and mistrust on his ability to discuss sensitive issues including religion. [Editor's note: Apparently, the decision of the therapist to make himself available as a real object, such as by discussing religious ideology, and feeding the patient's manifest need for the therapist's openness was too threatening. In this case, shared or similar religious background led to the patient's attempted idealization of the therapist which was at once satisfying to his inner need for "good" objects but also overwhelming. At that point, differences enphasized by the patient between his and the therapist's ideology served primarily to achieve distance, which also destroyed what little there was of any adequate therapeutic "holding" alliance.] His decision to guess at the patient's "major" problem and to then defend his own theology allowed the patient to project upon him the role of his father—a self-proclaimed expert who did not truly understand and could not accept doubters—so that he felt justified in leaving therapy. It would have been more helpful for the therapist to have asked the patient to explore what in the patient's view were the remaining problems and why he wished to pursue this, so that he could understand more clearly the issues at hand. In large part, the therapist lost sight of this because of his over-identification with the patient who was of similar age, from the same region of the country, and who, like the patient, continued to experience difficulty in relation to his conservative minister father.

Patients who initially idealize a religious therapist and then become too vulnerable to express the negative side of the transference can be even more difficult to treat. As an example (Case 7), a 24 year-old, single businessman and part-time seminary student was referred by a seminary professor to this author for help in focusing his career goals. The patient described being ridiculed and brutalized as a child in a working class family, escaping to boarding school because of his superior intelligence but losing the school's highest honor to a more favored older classmate. After a childhood and early adolescence marked by hurt and disappointment, he was much surprised by the positive attention he received in college. He became an evangelical Christian partly in response to the warmth and interest of a Christian campus organization and spent several months in a Christian commune before coming into conflict with its leader. At the time he came for treatment, he was beginning to experience disappointment with his conservative seminary and subsequently transferred to a more liberal one.

He typically began the early sessions by complimenting the therapist on how helpful his comments had been and then proceeded to discuss a list of his own insights concerning instances when he was misunderstood by others in graduate school, seminary, and in his work. While he rarely brought specifically religious questions into these sessions, he often indicated that the church was one place where he felt accepted. He appeared to appreciate a similar kind of acceptance from the therapist but after a few sessions began to arrive late and to accumulate an overdue balance. The therapist's attempts to explore the meaning of this behavior produced only concrete, defensive responses ("I'm always late — it has nothing to do with you"), and subsequently withdrawal from treatment. Under pressure, he eventually returned to discuss their different perceptions of the treatment and to work out a schedule for payment of his balance.

At this meeting, the patient said his understanding of their relationship had been one of his talking over "professional concerns" with a colleague and that he had begun to feel the therapist was attempting to manipulate and exploit him by attempting to discuss his feelings toward the therapist. In this case, the patient's view of the therapist as a helpful religious figure was designed to perpetuate the kind of uncritical acceptance of his behavior which he had enjoyed in the church but which was inappropriate to the psychotherapeutic situation. The therapist's inordinate wish to resuce this bright, ambitious, and in many ways appealing patient from traumatic experiences at the hands of family, schools, and conservative religious groups interfered with his professional ability to clarify early enough with the patient his expectations for the nature and goals of their work together. Also, the therapist had over-identified with the patient by virtue of his own similar experiences of feeling somewhat socially isolated as a child, competing to establish himself as a helping professional, and moving from a conservative to a more liberal religious affiliation. These uncontrolled factors made it difficult for him to recognize and address the patient's idealization of their relationship as unique and special by virtue of their common religious identification.

Another example (Case 8) illustrates how the same therapist dealt more effectively with a patient's presumption of specialness to and overfamiliarity with the therapist as a religious colleague. The patient was a 25 year-old single, white Baptist with two master's degrees but working at menial jobs. He was referred by his pastor for what the patient termed "issues of dependency." He described being an only child born to Catholic parents when they were in their mid-forties. He had always been concerned about pleasing his mother and attributed his being one hundred pounds overweight to both her unceasing attempts to feed him and his inability to say "no." At times, however, he was aware of resentment toward her for dominating both him and his father and for overprotecting him with automatic praise ("I could do no wrong").

He attended parochial school as a dutiful but nominal Catholic and became attracted during college to an active evangelical organization on campus. At that point, the patient joined the local Baptist church, eventually sharing an apartment with other students attending the church. While obtaining a master's degree in counselling in another state, he was advised by his supervisor to enter therapy because he appeared too "cocky" and was too presumptuous. This came as a shock to him, but he attended six sessions of therapy which he claimed were "helpful." Upon returning home, he spent another two years in an evangelical seminary, undecided about entering the ordained ministry or working as a pastoral counsellor. He elected treatment at a point when he had been unable to find work except as a night watchman. At the same time, he was disappointed by rejection by a woman who he had assumed would be more interested in him and was becoming concerned about remaining financially dependent on his parents through having to live at home.

He appeared somewhat anxious in sessions but also displayed a collegial, at times joking, overly familiar manner, using the therapist's first name, referring to other members of the church whom the therapist had seen, and expressing a future interest in the therapist's serving as his supervisor when he found clients of his own to counsel. It appeared that his sense of identity as both a helping professional and a diligent believer held a number of positive meanings for him, which intensified his inclination to identify with his religious therapist: use of his strengths, interest in people, a dependent connection with but the desire for some independence from his family, and a sense of value through involvement with a community of peers. He came to get help for his flagging self-esteem as he was becoming increasingly disappointed that his gifts and good will were not recognized by others as they had been by his mother at home.

Feeling that he was being asked to respond to the patient both as a member of the family (of faith) and as a professional with an established identity and insights which the patient wished to emulate, the therapist considered the following strategic options: 1) Directly discussing the patient's assumption of a first-name basis and other examples of overfamiliarity as inappropriate and an example of transference. 2) Adopting a counselling, quasi-supervisory role more consistent with the patient's own training as a religious counsellor. 3) Attempting to nurture a long-term alliance with the patient around his goal of greater independence and maturity from which to examine his behavior as it conflicted with this psychological and religious ideal.

The therapist followed the third approach and allowed the patient to bring in his own formulations as to why he was anxious or depressed at a particular point. For example, the focus turned to reality problems such as that the job market was simply too competitive, that psychiatric facilities did not want to hire mental health workers with religious training, or that women had not been straightforward with him about not wanting a romantic relationship. The therapist then gently encouraged the patient to explore other possible points of view (for example, that his employment problems had to do with his way of presenting himself and his limited experience might be equally important in his difficulty of finding work as his religious training, etc.), while also frustrating the patient's wish for approval of his own behavior and premature insights. By this time, however, sufficient trust had been established so that the patient could discuss his hurt feelings as a pattern of response he often had to others which led to his misreading their responses to him and being unduly disappointed as a result. In order to encourage this sense of trust, the therapist allowed the patient to use his first name and to ask for advice on occasion. In time such requests became less frequent.

This patient's overfamiliarity and sense of specialness in relation to the therapist had childhood origins but were also fed by his religious expectations for fellow believers to share informally as a family and by his identification with the independence and respectability of the therapist as a helping professional. The therapist, at first, often felt annoyed by the patient's personal and religious style but shared enough common ground with the patient to be able to accept his

wish for specialness and eventually to examine it as part of the therapeutic work. Over the next two years, with appointments every two-
to-three weeks, the patient obtained work as a mental health
attendant, then also a chaplain, lost 70 pounds, and married a member of the church.

In most of the preceding examples, the patients assumed,
without explicit discussion of the issue, that the therapist shared
their religious beliefs. At times, however, patients question their
therapist's religious beliefs and make these an overt issue in the treatment. As an example (Case 9), a 25 year-old, unmarried college student came for treatment for chronic depression and bulimia. She
had begun to attend a conservative Christian church with her boyfriend but became disillusioned with the church when their relationship broke up. She looked for a religious therapist because she felt
that she "should" trust God and attend church but that her resentments and depression made it impossible for her to do so. Further
exploration revealed that her attitude toward God paralleled her attitude toward her family, her bulimia self-help group, and the therapist. She resented God's expectations as unreachable and arbitrary,
as many of her family's expectations of her as a child had been, but
felt inadequate and guilty for not meeting these expectations. In the
case of God's expectations, she felt expected either to believe or to
not bother to attend church—the course she most often took. Her
perfectionistic tendencies and fears of rejection impaired her ability
to question the perceived expectations of others (for example, that
she be a sensitive listener at all times in order to be considered a
friend), and to accept her own limitations.

After some time she began to question the therapist about his religious standards (Did he believe sex before marriage was wrong?
What about abortion? Could one be a Christian and hold liberal political views?). The therapist regarded the emergence of this questioning attitude as evidence that the patient now felt more able to
question beliefs that she previously had felt obligated to accept.
However, perhaps also feeling a need to defend the faith, he responded with some of his own incomplete answers to these questions, hoping to offer a model of serious consideration of such
questions. The patient could not accept the therapist's perspectives

on some issues (e.g., that biblical statements about sex before marriage have practical reasons behind them and represent a statement of the ideal rather than arbitrary and absolute prohibitions), and tended to argue with him about them. At the same time, she was reassured when the therapist did not reject her for disagreeing with him. In response to her question about whether he believed a Christian could approve of abortion, he shared with her a publication examining the issues from a Christian perspective that was neither exclusively "pro-life" nor "pro-choice." She responded with surprise that "such people existed." After this point, contentious or dogmatic argumentation about religious issues became less a focus of treatment.

The patient continued to complain at times that she missed a close relationship with God but was unwilling to return to a church which seemed intolerably rigid and conservative. When the therapist asked about the possibility of visiting other types of churches as a way of resolving this conflict, she said she had not done so because she "wouldn't know where to start," and feared this could threaten her familiar if ambivalently held beliefs. She then wondered what the therapist's opinion was. The therapist considered withholding his own religious perspective until they had more fully examined her reason for asking, but he decided that at this point in therapy his silence might lead to her withdrawal out of feeling rejected, deprived, and possibly controlled. The approach of sharing in a nonjudgmental way of some of his own religious perspectives as an example of the availability of other points of view actually provided her with novel experience. Their subsequent discussion of this experience allowed her to see that her tendency to argue about or feel burdened by their religious differences was perhaps an example of the way in which her emotional set tended to deprive her of opportunities for growth and support. From here, the focus returned naturally to more directly psychotherapeutic concerns such as the operation and origin of this tendency in relation to her family, her friends, and her career.

In this case, the therapist's appreciation for the meaning of the patient's request to know something about his religious beliefs, combined with a heightened awareness of the need to explore the patient's motives for needing such knowledge, allowed him to respond in a way that fostered the therapy through an enhanced sense of openness and shared humanity. Sharing his own religious beliefs was much less helpful in Case 6 because it led to avoidance of an important clinical issue and evoked an unhealthy pattern of interactions with other authority figures in the patient's life. Both examples illustrate the importance of an awareness of the meaning of discussing religious issues, both for the therapist and the patient. If sharing personal religious perspectives seems at odds with what the patient needs from the therapist, the therapist can consider other options: e.g., to share literature representing alternative points of view, as in Cases 5 and 9, or to help the patient to explore alternative sources of religious support and guidance. The following two cases exemplify this second approach.

A first-year seminary student (Case 10) brought to the therapist concerns about whether he could legitimately aspire to become a pastor, given certain perplexing doubts, anxieties, and past failings. The therapist, to whom the patient had been referred by his pastor and who had helped the patient over the preceding two years through similar periods of anxiety in relation to other decisions, encouraged him to view the issue as another instance of performance anxiety which he usually had been able to master with time and support. However, he also encouraged the patient to further explore his doubts with his pastor and an advisor at the seminary for their comments on his performance and his worthiness to represent the church. They would be the ones best suited to lend a religious perspective to his worries and doubts. In this case the therapist did not pursue the religious aspects of this decision for two reasons. First, in order to convey his expectation that the patient was able to make reasonable decisions in an area where he had some competence. Second, in order to reinforce what appeared to be an understanding and supportive relationship between the patient and his pastor as a more appropriate basis for identification in the patient's struggle with religious issues.

Another patient (Case 11), a 34 year-old man with a long history of drug abuse, was diagnosed with cancer while serving a jail term for stealing. He requested psychiatric help at the cancer center because of a nightmare in which Jesus and Satan, in the form of a rat and a pig, were fighting over his soul. When he awoke, he felt that he was in Hell and that suicide was the only way out. He managed to stop himself at the last minute from carrying out the suicide. In a tearful turmoil during the next two days, he described feeling guilty for the first time in his twenty years of crime, writing down many of his experiences in the form of a confession. He had not attended church since parochial school but reported that certain religious literature he had obtained now "made sense" to him for the first time.

The therapist explored with him the meaning of this experience in terms of the re-evaluation of his life occasioned by the recent stresses of his imprisonment, his cancer, and the recent suicide of his best friend. The therapist also discussed with the prison staff ways of providing the patient adequate support and opportunity to talk and write during the crisis. He also encouraged the patient's interest in speaking with a priest about his sense of guilt and his wish to realign the priorities in his life. In this case, the patient did not envision the therapist as a religious figure, having already identified another source of religious help in the priest. Thus, the therapist attempted to help the patient examine why he felt so guilty (in terns of what standards he held up for himself and whether these were realistic), but did not feel that he was in a position to offer the deeper sense of forgiveness and basis for faith for which the patient now searched.

DIRECTIVE RELIGIOUS COUNSELLING
IN PSYCHOTHERAPY

The question of to what degree a therapist of the same or any faith should engage in religious counselling with patients will be answered differently by psychotherapists with different personal styles. Therapists with a more giving or directive style may use shared religious language to achieve ends which they view as desirable from both a religious as well as psychological point of view.

For example (Case 12), a 24 year-old conservative Protestant physical therapist sought out a Christian psychiatrist because of difficulty choosing between two physicians she was dating. When she felt criticized by the therapist in his exploration of her difficulty in sustaining intimate relationships, she developed panic attacks. She then arranged to see instead a younger Christian colleague who emphasized more her strengths and previous lack of support for them in her family (which had become more supportive since several family members had become evangelical Christians). The second therapist felt that the patient identified him positively with her older brother, also a physician, to whom she looked for guidance, and he made use of this transference to offer suggestions of a religious and psychological nature: that she find a "spiritual mother" or female mentor to help her growth, that she pray for others as well as for her own healing, and that she consider some of the religious insights which he had found helpful in his own life. She warmed to this approach and her symptoms improved. When this psychiatrist left the area six months later, she herself moved to a more urban area and began more work with this author. With this third therapist, she continued to maintain that she would not become romantically involved with a man who was not a "born-again" Christian, although she did find a less conservative church which she attended less often, felt more independent in her career and with her friends, and was no longer seeking such active religious or psychological guidance from a therapist. Instead she seemed to want availability and understanding from a third therapist whom she saw on a monthly then on an as needed basis. In this case, the use of shared religious language and concepts by the second therapist had been helpful in re-establishing the patient's trust in him and in herself during a crisis time. His style of religious and therapeutic approach was both relatively directive but also informed by an understanding of the needs of the patient and of his meaning to her as a transference figure. Had he not moved away form the area and had he continued to see her as she became more self-confident and less involved in their conservative church, one can speculate whether their relationship would have changed to resemble her relationship to the third therapist (in which neither religious nor active psychological direction played an important role), or whether ambivalence toward him as a directive authority figure connected with his directive religious style would have eventually made it difficult for them to work together.

CHANGES IN PATIENTS' RELIGIOSITY

Changes and development in the process of patients' religious lives occur frequently and provide an important opportunity for therapists to understand and help with the development of both the patients' inner life and the quality of their relationship to others. A number of patients discussed in this chapter came to me as a religious therapist at a point in their lives when they felt their church was no longer able to meet their needs. In the case of the more disturbed patients (Cases 1 and 11), this was due to their unusual emotional needs and unrealistic expectations. Psychotherapy and sometimes the structure of another institution were needed to render these patients capable of receiving much of what the church had to offer. In a second group of patients struggling to become independent from controlling families and conflict-inducing religious backgrounds (Cases 5, 6, 7, and 9), ambivalence toward both of these interfered with the development of a therapeutic alliance and with the patients' ability to participate in a religious community. It is easier in the therapy of such patients for the therapist to become involved in complicating and potentially distorting interactions especially along the lines of both parties' different motivations for religious beliefs and needs. Psychotherapy directed to this issue helped some of these patients to develop more open attitudes toward their faith, but few returned to active participation in church during their therapy. A third group of patients with an active relationship with the church and the therapist (Cases 2, 3, 4, 8, 10, 12) made use of both in ways which were at times complementary and on occasion collaborative.

Differences between my religious beliefs and my patients' religious beliefs within the same tradition have exerted greatest influence in my practice of psychotherapy at points where the patient has felt religiously obligated to judge his behavior more harshly than I (Case 9). From a psychotherapeutic point of view, I generally take the position that moral judgments of behavior are less helpful than and sometimes interfere with attempts to understand its origins and meanings. Patients who have difficulty suspending judgment in this way (Cases 4, 5, 6, 9) are likely to question the nature and strength of my beliefs. If they discover that from a religious point of view I am inclined to emphasize God's grace (forgiveness) over judgment (in the sense of assigning blame, which I prefer to leave to God), they may suspect me of being in favor of vacuous relativism and perhaps question in turn the moral underpinnings of psychotherapy (Cases 5, 6, and 9).

A final example (Case 13) illustrates a patient's fear of considering more "liberal" religious perspectives than those familiar to her even though she found her conservative church rigid and unsatisfying. A 32 year-old part-time graduate student and mother of a young, physically impaired child was referred to me by her internist, a member of her church, because of increasing symptoms of anxiety and depression. The patient was the youngest and least academically successful of the three children in an upper middle class achievement-oriented family. She viewed herself as unattractive and insecure as a child and was also fearful as an adult of being rejected as inadequate. This, despite the fact that she was bright, verbal, and accomplished in several areas. During her divorce after three years of marriage to an alcoholic artist, she became an active Christian through a woman for whom she worked as a homemaker. Although at times resentful of God for the burden of responsibility she felt, she continued to regard God as the most important sustaining influence in her life.

She came for therapy two years after moving with her second husband and their child from the country to the city so that they could both attend graduate school. Several stresses seemed important at the time of referral: the demands of caring for their physically impaired child, a heightened sense of social and academic competition in a new setting, less time with her husband, and an inability to find a church in which both husband and wife felt comfortable. When I asked about their search for another church, she asked what church I attended. I simply gave her the name of my church (in a closely related denomination). She responded that she could not accept a woman as a pastor—I had not mentioned the sex of my pastor—because her interpretation of the Bible did not permit this. She went on to explain her fear that a less thanliteral interpretation of the Bible on such points would undermine the basis of belief in "the promises of God," as well as in other doctrines which some might consider less important. It seemed clear that her fear of losing the valuable support of these promises (in particular, that God would accept and love her despite her inadequacies) made her reluctant to question even apparently unrelated doctrines of the conservative church which had brought her this sense of support. I acknowledged that it can be risky to choose which doctrines to believe, but I did not press the point that it also is sometimes necessary or helpful to do so. At the same time, I hoped that if she chose further to discuss her religious struggles with me, perhaps as a psychotherapist who understood her anxieties as well as the benefits of positive religious experience, I could help her understand the influence of her long-standing fears of rejection on her ability to remain open to helpful possibilities in this as well as in other areas of her life. This approach led to a productive treatment relationship.

In summary, I have offered several examples which demonstrate some of the ways in which sensitivity to the interplay of religious and psychological issues can enhance the perspective of both patient and therapist on the process of psychotherapy as neither a simple technical exercise nor a substitute for faith but a complex human enterprise involving the whole person.

REFERENCES

Allport, G.W. *The Individual and His Religion*. New York: Macmillan Company, 1950.

Apolito, A. Psychoanalysis and religion. *American Journal of Psychoanalysis*, 1970, *30*, 115-126.

Cohen, R.J. & Smith, F.S. Socially reinforced obsessing: Etiology of disorder in a Christian Scientist. *Journal of Consulting and Clinical Psychology*, 1976, *44*, 142-144.

Freud, S. *The Future of an Illusion*. New York: W.W. Norton, 1928.

Halleck, S.L. Discussion of "socially reinforced obsessing." *Journal of Consulting and Clinical Psychology*, 1976, *44*, 146-147.

James, W. *The Varieties of Religious Experience*. New York: Longmans, Green and Co., 1902.

Levin, T.M. & Zegans, L.S. Adolescent identity crisis and religious conversion.

British Journal of Medical Psychology, 1974, *47*, 73-82.

London, P. Psychotherapy for religious neuroses? Comments on Cohen and Smith. *Journal of Consulting and Clinical Psychology*, 1976, *44*, 145-146.

McLemore, C.W. & Court, J.H. Religion and psychotherapy — ethics, civil liberties, and clinical savvy: A critique. *Journal of Consulting and Clinical Psychology*, 1977, *45*, 1172-1175.

Pattison, E.M. Social and psychological aspects of religion in psychotherapy. *Journal of Nervous and Mental Disease*, 1966, *141*, 586-597.

Peteet, J.R. Issues in the treatment of religious patients. *American Journal of Psychotherapy*, 1981, *35*, 564-565.

Pruyser, P.W. Assessment of the patient's religious attitudes in the psychiatric case study. *Bulletin of the Menninger Clinic*, 1971, *35*, 272-291.

Rieff, P. *Freud: The Mind of the Moralist*. London: Methuen and Co., 1959.

Rizzuto, A.M. Object relations and the formation of the image of God. *British Journal of Medical Psychology*, 1974, *47*, 83-99.

Spero, M.H. Clinical aspects of religion as neurosis. *American Journal of Psychoanalysis*, 1976, *36*, 361-365.

Spero, M.H. Countertransference in religious therapists of religious patients. *American Journal of Psychotherapy*, 1981, *35*, 565-576.

Chapter 4

RELIGIOUS VALUES AND THE THERAPEUTIC ALLIANCE, OR "HELP ME, PSYCHOLOGIST; I HATE YOU, RABBI!"

PAUL KAHN, Ph.D.

WHEN a patient comes to a psychotherapist with knowledge that the therapist is also a member of the clergy, a number of clinically important issues arise. For instance, it is generally recognized that psychoanalytically-oriented psychotherapy is best conducted in a relationship which respects the limits of the therapeutic "frame." It is generally unwarranted to allow the client too many opportunities to relate to the therapist's personal life or convictions. Maintenance of the therapist's relative anonymity is a significant component in the establishment of the therapeutic alliance (Langs, 1978, p. 192). Knowledge that one's psychotherapist is a clergyman and the system of values the patient perceives as related to that position may engender numerous misalliance problems involving transference and countertransference issues. In addition, discussion of religious values as they relate to the therapeutic process is likely to occur and this may involve the therapist in aspects of his own identity which typically are not subjected during training to self-analysis, or which are conflictual for the therapist. But when such knowledge is unavoidable, the therapist is presented with the challenge of deciding what therapeutic approach and techniques should be used, allowing the therapy to proceed to a successful conclusion.

The present paper illustrates this specific clinical situation. The patient to be discussed came to me for therapeutic help and knew that I was a rabbi in the community in addition to my professional career as a psychologist. While a minority of my patients are aware of my rabbinical position, this knowledge has rarely played the significant role that it did in the following case.

INITIAL PRESENTATION OF THE
DUAL ROLE PROBLEMATIC

When Irving entered my office for the first time, he appeared familiar although at first I could not place him. He was 30 years old, single, and unable to tolerate his loneliness. He proceeded to inform me that he felt he needed to talk to a psychologist and that he chose me since he knew me as a rabbi in the community and in past years had a few times attended services in my synagogue.

Irving's religiosity can be described as modern orthodox. He came from an irreligious Jewish home and became orthodox during his adolescent years under the influence of a charismatic Hasidic teacher. He very soon related a series of tragic events having to do with significant personal losses that had left him extremely lonely (these will not be detailed in order to safeguard the patient's identity). He described an intense need for companionship and sexual relations and also of having established a sexual relationship with a young lady by the name of Shirley. He described her as an exceptionally beautiful girl who was not as religious as he but who wanted to marry him. Since orthodox Judaism does not permit physical sexual behavior prior to marriage, Irving was now experiencing a religious dilemma and did not know what to do.

Thus began a psychotherapeutic relationship that lasted for three years. A rather dependent and emotionally labile young man, probably a hysterical personality, Irving presented difficult but not atypical therapeutic challenges from the standpoint of psychodynamics. However, the intertwining of neurotic problems within the context of the patient's orthodox Jewish practices and values presented the therapist, himself an orthodox Jew, with unique transference and countertransference challenges. This case study focuses upon these latter issues and only secondarily upon the more or less ordinary dynamics of the therapeutic process and an understanding of Irving himself. I will attempt to clarify the motivations of the patient, the problems they presented for the therapist, the feelings of the therapist, and the resolutions effected.

I begin with comments on the initial session whose full significance, as usual, emerged in retrospect towards the end of the therapeutic process. The major motivation behind Irving's seeking out a religious therapist with dual roles was to obtain license for his sexual liaison. At a later point it became clear that Irving from the start was somewhat aware that for him the prospect of marrying Shirley would entail abandoning his religiosity, a development that at one level he welcomed. The "bait" for eliciting this allowance would be the grounds of his mental health, his loneliness and suffering, his irrevocable psychological "needs" pitted against the norms of his religious beliefs. He therefore split his experience of the therapist in two: psychologist and rabbi. As psychologist, I would be expected to provide license on the basis of mental health considerations to show an appreciation for his psychological needs as superordinate to his religious obligations. Once offered, such appreciation would have for this particular patient the power of a rabbinical dispensation (*heter*), drawn from my second role as rabbi, to somehow suspend religious obligations in the interests of mental health. Were such allowances to be denied, Irving could attack my psychological sophistication and at the same time be angry at the "old-fashioned rabbi" for his lack of understanding.

Placing the therapist in this trap replicated the dual image and conflicting needs Irving felt regarding his own internalized father-figures (primarily that of his natural father and his Hasidic teacher). I initially could not completely foresee the dynamic meaning of this trap and was presented with the problem of how to respond both as psychologist and rabbi. I felt puzzled and uncomfortable. The resolution I offered was to not answer his questions directly but rather to suggest that further discussion was indicated to explore whether the problems the patient presented needed to be dealt with psychotherapeutically. After further discussion we agreed to continue sessions on a weekly basis.

During the beginning therapeutic phase of the next few months, Irving began to articulate and understand his marked dependency and intense anger in response to non-gratification of his dependency needs. These feelings had been problematic since childhood and were currently adversely affecting his ability to function on his job. This was particularly noted in relation to his bosses (authority figures) toward whom he would react with resentment when he felt unappreciated. During these early months of therapy, his maladaptive behavior at work began to show some improvement.

Irving gradually began to elaborate upon a more bothersome problem involving a compulsion to attend pornographic movies and buy pornographic magazines. His compulsive involvement in pornography appeared to be associated with an eroticization of his core problem (dependency plus anger), insofar as his interest in erotically stimulating females was associated with oral dependency while his demeaning attitude "punished" them for not loving him and taking care of him. He eventually presented his pornographic interests within the context of the transference relationship, passively seeking both support and forgiveness from a therapist from whom he hoped to receive limitless love, care, and concern. This I found relatively easy to handle therapeutically, primarily through interpretation and generally helping the patient gain insight into the meanings of his uncontrollable interest in pornography. When indicated, I interpreted the negative and positive aspects of the transference in the same perspective. I encouraged Irving to continue therapeutic work.

EMERGENCE OF THE
NEUROSIS-RELIGION INTERFACE

During the following month, Irving returned to the issue of his ongoing relationship with Shirley. It appeared that again he was seeking to have me validate his relationship with her. Again, my problem was how to respond. I was increasingly aware that my own religious values were influencing my feelings. Insofar as Irving's continued sexual liaison with Shirley compromised his orthodox commitments, I felt as a rabbi the urge to "do something about it," to comment, perhaps to moralize. Nevertheless, I resolved to focus on clarifying Irving's *neurotic* needs regarding his relationship with Shirley. These included feelings of dependency, compensation for a sense of failure (sexual as well as otherwise) during adolescence, oedipal issues, confused relationships with a nurturing mother and a sexually provocative sister, and oedipal rage toward an autocratic and demanding father.

Irving's internalized father image had evolved from a combination of a competitive, domineering father who strongly disapproved of Irving's becoming religious during adolescence and various rabbinic figures who in his late adolescence and early adult life continued the pattern of not gratifying Irving's dependency needs and made domineering attempts to control his life. A third element was the internalization of a deity that caused him great personal tragedy during adult life (the death of a female love-object) and was seen in part as the embodiment of all previous negative authority figures.

His intense attraction to Shirley appeared to involve his acting-out feelings and fantasies related to internalized female figures (see the above discussion regarding his nurturing mother and sexually provocative sister) as well as feelings related to internalized father figures. The latter involved proving his adequacy in relation to his demeaning and castrating father as well as directing anger at and establishing autonomy from rabbinic figures and God himself. Later in therapy, from understandings gained through the transference relationship, it became more clear how Irving was splitting the therapist as a transference object into an idealized, kindly psychologist from whom he expected continual support and guidance, and the rabbi/father who was harsh, ungiving, and controlling, and towards whom he could re-direct his anger and intense disappointment. A basic issue that evolved in therapy was conflict between the gratification of dependency needs and growing up. Ongoing anger was felt towards the therapist for "forcing" him to be mature. In this regard, the non-gratifying therapist could be perceived as the actively depriving rabbi. Experiencing the "badness" of the therapist as the therapist *qua* rabbi allowed Irving to protect the "good" aspects of the therapist *qua* nurturing, idealized psychologist. While at times these transference distortions were difficult to handle, they presented material for good therapeutic work. It was becoming clear why Irving's relationship with Shirley had become a central therapeutic issue, and why transference and countertransference issues had to be confronted.

RELIGIOUS CONFLICTS
IN THE COUNTERTRANSFERENCE

During subsequent therapeutic sessions, Irving continued to be preoccupied with Shirley. His doubts regarding their relationship increased as he reported disturbed qualities of her behavior. Interestingly, it was only after Shirley's own psychiatrist recommended that she and Irving terminate their relationship that Irving began to speak of being "altruistically" motivated to marry her precisely becauce of her psychiatric problems. After some hesitancy, I decided to adopt a somewhat more active posture, highlighting for Irving Shirley's apparent psychopathology. After a few sessions, Irving accused me of being biased in my position regarding the entire issue and that I was being too religiously-oriented.

I vividly recall experiencing conflict during this stage, a conflict between different professional approaches as well as conflict between religious and therapeutic values. On one hand, I have a strong professional commitment to the preservation of a relatively passive attitude, thereby challenging the patient to make decisions and maturely confront life's choices. On the other hand, it appeared that Irving was in need of reality confrontation and perhaps a greater degree of support to accomplish what I considered necessary therapeutic movement. Within myself, however, doubts lingered whether adopting this more active position was motivated solely by therapeutic reasons, or was I responding to my religious values and rabbinical role? I believed I was making rationally valid treatment decisions, but it was undeniable that the change to more active intervention also satisfied my religious values. Was I truly responding to the psychological conflicts and fixations represented by Irving's behavior or merely to its religious impropriety, or was there a way to respond to both? In so doing, would I lose my professional posture and become primarily a rabbinic counselor? My reactions were associated with a tendency to feel guilty for feelings as if they were actions, a reaction which I could accept as clearly non-logical. On the other hand, perhaps my guilt and unease were appropriate reactions to therapeutic errors and that I was indeed completely misinterpreting the meaning of and motivation behind my actions. With the attachment of these latter feelings to my rational judgment, I tended to doubt the cognitive clarity of my decision, especially as Irving proceeded to attack me precisely on this issue, as noted above in his accusation of my being biased and too religiously-oriented.

I responded to these reactions first by continually rechecking the validity of my therapeutic approach both in terms of material being presented as well as my own feelings. Second, I tried to keep my comments as nonintrusive as possible, thereby maintaining Irving's responsibility for choice and growth and not creating transference-countertransference havoc. This was especially important in Irving's case in view of the centrality in his overall pattern of adjustment of dependency issues and his fear of growing up. For me to have become markedly directive would have been to withhold from Irving the potential growth-evoking experience of therapy. In addition, a directive approach may have engendered rage previously felt towards controlling parental and authority figures. Such rage would undoubtedly complicate productive transference material insofar as Irving's feelings would then have to be understood partly as a realistic reaction to the therapist's intrusiveness and activeness, and could disrupt the therapeutic alliance. As an example of my nonintrusive approach, in taking note of Shirley's pathological behavior and its effect upon Irving, I did not specifically recommend that he terminate their relationship, but rather helped him to confront the difficulties of their relationship. For me, the dilemma continued to be whether I was therapeutically aiding Irving to confront reality or manipulating him to concede to an *a priori* religious commitment.

RESOLUTION OF SOME
COUNTERTRANSFERENCE ISSUES

Irving remained in treatment for an additional two years. During this time, an interesting number of changes took place both in my own orientation as well as in Irving's behavior. I happened at that time to be personally involved in a number of professional discussion groups exploring the relationship between Jewish religious-legal norms of ethical responsibility and the psychotherapeutic process. An increasing sense of moral responsibility toward my patient's behavior indicated to me that I could not simplistically ignore religious values during psychotherapy. This conviction impelled me to more intensively study the possible effects, including negative effects, that such "value intervention" might have. Directive and perhaps even manipulative injection of my values into the therapeutic process in fact would not result in fulfillment of moral responsibility because this approach would probably not achieve any lasting internalization of such values on the patient's part. In a sense, the patient was neither psychologically nor morally prepared for this. The result of an injection of values may have well led to an oppositional reaction in therapy or even to the patient's bolting from therapy. It seemed, instead, that consistent application of standard therapeutic technique would itself be the best method for helping the patient to accept mature responsibility for his own behavior. But in doing so, the therapist must be alert to not allow the patient to perceive silence or other passive behavior as sanction or encouragement for inappropriate behavior (see Kahn, 1983).

I was once provided with an example of such misperception of silence when an orthodox Jewish adolescent patient told me that he had stopped wearing a skullcap in opposition to a controlling father. His movement toward psychological independence appeared otherwise appropriate and I was hesitant to intervene at that point with a comment on this specific act of religious behavior. No further discussion of the issue followed and I forgot about the event. Months later he told me how he had gone to eat in a non-Kosher restaurant. At that point I noted that such action appeared to be a rather radical step for him. He countered by saying, "But you said it was OK for me to stop being religious." Surprised, I asked when I had so suggested. He responded that this was his interpretation of my non-reaction to his earlier report of no longer wearing his skullcap. To return to the main discussion, while the initial task of confronting the role of values in psychotherapy provided the therapist some conceptual complications, a deeper grasp of the therapeutic process also emerged which provided me with a greater sense of assuredness.

Irving made considerable progress during the course of therapy. In his personal life, he began to work more responsibly and experienced less conflict relating to authority figures. He terminated his relationship with Shirley, began to date, and eventually married an orthodox though somewhat rigid woman. Through therapeutic growth, he gained control over his compulsive involvement with pornography. However, shortly after his marriage, marital problems began to develop. He was increasingly angry at his wife, whose demanding behavior was conflicting with his own dependency needs. (Eventually it was recommended that the wife seek therapy.) Irving had told his wife about his previous sexual behavior, about Shirley, and his past history with pornography. He had expected his wife to both accept his previous maladaptive behavior as well as compliment him on his successful struggles to improve. Unfortunately for him, his wife reacted with abhorence and rejection. This sets the stage for the description of the following session.

Irving related his puzzlement regarding his wife's contradictory reaction to sexual relations. During the week before she would go to the *mikveh*˙, Irving would seduce her. Although such behavior is religiously proscribed, his wife's reaction would be quite passionate. Yet, after she would return from the *mikveh*, all ensuing sexual relations were marked by coldness on her part.

I had a number of personal reactions to the above material. Even though I developed some hypotheses regarding his wife's psychological needs and conflicts, I decided that an interpretation of her sexual behavior was not yet indicated. Moreover, I was well aware that be-

---

˙A ritual bath into which orthodox Jewish women immerse themselves a week after termination of menstruation, thereby allowing the sexual relations to commence. Sexual relations and other forms of phycial intimacy are not allowed from the onset of menstruation until after immersion into the *mikveh*.

fore me sat an orthodox Jew describing a pattern of religiously forbidden behavior. I decided to wait and listen. After a while, Irving
spontaneously expressed full knowledge of the forbidden nature of
his behavior and was actually quite precise in describing its
stringency. It occurred to me that I could not have added any factual
information regarding his behavior that he did not already know. I
did not interrupt. Irving then appeared to shift topics and began
talking about Shirley and then about his former interest in pornography. At first I was concerned that I might miss the opportunity of
making a useful intervention regarding the first issue. But I continued to remain silent. When he finished talking about pornography, I
made some tentative inquiries which provided me with sufficient
material to offer a major interpretation. I suggested that because of
his hurt and anger at his wife for not accepting his sexually "deviant"
past, he seduced her at a forbidden time thereby transforming her
into a deviant, making her also a sexual "sinner" like himself. (The
reason for her readiness for such seduction indicated her own sexual
conflicts, but no interpretation of her behavior was offered.) After
his wife went to the *mikveh*, she retaliated, punishing him for what he
had done.

Irving accepted the interpretation and proceeded to react to it
with a changed emotional quality. He no longer spoke in his charac-
terisitic charged, emotionally pressured manner. Rather, he spoke in
a solemn, thoughtful manner, with a quality of inner peace. He now
realized how much of the situation was a result of his own actions,
and thereby the degree to which he himself could effect positive
change.

Trgratent was terminated a short while after the previously reported session. Behavioral maladaptation relating to religious values
continued to be dealt with constructively within the framework of a
therapeutic alliance. In reviewing Irving's treatment, I was impressed with the ability of good, classical therapeutic technique to
fulfill both my professional goals as well as my religious obligation to
be concerned about the quality of a patient's religious behavior.
Directive, critical "rebuke" typical of a pastoral approach would have
been ineffective at best, disasterous at worse. By waiting, understanding, and interpreting—by enabling the patient to reconcile on

his own the internal tensions and conflicts which motivated his particular form of inappropriate religious expression — therapeutic as well as religious obligations had been fulfilled. Furthermore, the splitting of the psychotherapist into gratifying psychologist and rejecting rabbi had been resolved by addressing the underlying dynamics of this split in the patient's identifications and religious ideals. My own splitting in this regard, based in my dual role and the patient's perception and attempted manipulation of these roles, had been repaired and I became a single entity confident in Irving's ability to maturely deal with life's problems. He had in time become a less dependent and less angry person with a minimal amount of neurotic behavioral manifestations in his interpersonal and religious life.

REFERENCES

Kahn, P. Psychotherapy and the commandment to reprove. *Proceedings of the Association of Orthodox Jewish Scientists*, 1983, *7*, 37-50.
Langs, R. *Technique in Transition*. New York: Jason Aronson, 1978.

Chapter 5

THE RELIGIOUS IDENTITY
OF THE PSYCHOANALYST
AS AN ISSUE IN PSYCHOANALYSIS

DAVID A. HALPERIN, M.D.
and
IRA SCHARFF, M.S.W., A.C.S.W.

GENERAL ISSUES

THE identity of the psychoanalyst and the manner in which it affects his relationships with his patients remains a matter of continuing scrutiny and concern. The extent to which the personal belief systems, attitudes, and concerns of the psychoanalyst alter the character and quality of treatment as well as its direction and the issues raised during the course of treatment, or even its ultimate efficacy, are relevant and meaningful questions even if they are unanswerable in an absolute sense. The importance of these questions is reflected in continuing discussion of the criteria which are subsumed under the label of the "good match" between psychoanalyst and analysand. For example, there has been considerable examination of the extent to which biases grounded in gender or sexual orientation affect the process of psychoanalysis (see Lester, 1983). A

The first part of this chapter was written by David A. Halperin and the second part by Halperin and Ira Scharff. The authors express appreciation to Patricia Heldman, M.D. for her thoughtful suggestions and kind critique of this paper.

similar concern has been expressed over the possibility of fulfilling analytic work when a racial difference exists between psychoanalyst and analysand (Goldensohn, 1981; Teichner, 1981). This paper will explore the importance of the psychoanalyst's religious identity as it may affect the course of psychodynamically-oriented psychotherapy.

As has been noted elsewhere, psychotherapists are often prone to consider the intense religious concerns of their patients with either intense skepticism or at the very least as being strongly suggestive of psychopathology (Halperin, 1983). A therapist's discomfort with his own or his patient's religiosity was eloquently expressed by Freud in his preface to the Hebrew edition of *Totem and Taboo* (1930):

> No reader of (the Hebrew version of) this book will find it easy to put himself in the emotional position of an author who is ignorant of the language of holy writ, who is completely estranged from the religion of his fathers — as well as from every other religion — and who cannot take a share in nationalist ideals, but who has never repudiated his people, who feels that he is in his essential nature a Jew and who has no desire to alter that nature. If the question were put to him: "Since you have abandoned all these common characteristics of your countrymen, what is there left to you that is Jewish?" he would reply: "A very great deal and probably its very essence."

In a sense, the impact of the psychoanalyst's religious identity, and the possibility that psychoanalysis, generally, simply might be regarded by the non-Jewish world as a species of Jewish messianism, underlay much of the complex relationship between Freud and Jung (Bettelheim, 1983) and much of their conflict (Bloom, 1982). Within the contemporary clinical context, the increasing rapprochement between psychodynamic psychotherapy and the intense religious conviction of its clientele has been evidenced by the growth of programs within major agencies such as the Jewish Board of Family and Children's Services of New York and the Westchester Jewish Community Services in which the insights afforded by religious tradition and supported by religious practice are treated with respect rather than disdain.

CLINICAL ILLUSTRATIONS

The interaction between the Jewish psychoanalyst and the non-Jewish patient may raise the issue of the analyst's Jewish identity in widely differing ways. The following examples illustrate this complex interweaving of idealization, expectation, and transference.

> (1) A black mental health professional commenting on her psychoanalyst, "I was really disappointed when he told me that he planned to see me for my session on the Day of Atonement. I'd been looking forward to having a day off...."

Here, the patient is expressing her confusion when confronted with her analyst's alienation from his own religious background. This professional from a rigid and religiously committed background expected all Jews to be the People of the Book and any divergence was regarded with a mixture of cynicism ("he won't cancel a session for anything....") and relief.

> (2) An Irish-American professional asserts:
> "I resent your charging me for a rescheduled group session. After all, the session had been rescheduled to take into account your holiday (the session was originally scheduled for the first night of Passover). Sometimes, I think your insistence and determination to be paid reflects your background."

This patient, an Irish-American financial expert, is directly expressing his resentment towards the analyst for his being Jewish and also for his not being the father whom he simultaneously idealized and denigrated. The patient was encouraged to explore his competitive feelings towards Jews and his own need to disavow personal characteristics which he preferred to see as specifically Jewish such as a concern over financial matters. Subsequently, he was able to pursue a former employer for past wages and to recover the substantial sums which he had previously considered bad debts.

Consider some other examples.

> (3) "I wish you'd gone up in smoke." An outburst uttered by a patient during the course of a group session and directed towards an obsessive and controlling group member who was a Holocaust survivor.

(4) The following peroration was delivered by an Irish-American professional in the textile field as she was discussing her summer, during which time she was sharing a house in the very Jewishly populated community of Westhampton:

"I'm consistently angry at Jews. I'm sick and tired of being in a Jewish world. I'm tired of it. I'd like to be in a Gentile world. Everything in this city is so oriented toward Judaism. My summer house. The house is very Jewish. It does get to me. Their talking about these Jewish matters. It's very annoying to me in a certain way. Next year, I'd like to get into a Gentile house. I'm tired of it in a certain way. I'd like to have more Gentile experience. There is a woman in the house, E. (her Jewish housemate), who's my ideal. She's like Zsa Zsa Gabor. She's short, pretty, very stylish and she knows her way around men. I really like and respect her. She's funny and understated. I modeled myself after her at a party....E. is this idealized woman. She's on a pedestal. She became friends with B. They're both Jewish. I like these people. They're very nice...."

These comments were amplified in a later session:

"The Jewish family is very close. I feel very sad that I don't have that in my life. I think Sheila is really involved in her family. She's very accepting of Sheldon. Sheldon is very dogmatic and ruminates a lot. But, Sheila's very tolerant of his eccentricities.

"I'm not tolerant of B's eccentricities. I don't think he'll change. Actually, I can see that there's a part of me that really doesn't want to get involved....

"Actually, I resent Sheldon because he takes Sheila away from me. It makes me very sad that he takes Sheila away from me and she's the only person I've ever met who is available for my type of friendship. Sheldon—it's awful that he has to be so involved with Sheila.

"It's my anger towards my mother. She never cared at all about how I looked. There were so many children and she said that she was always involved in them...."

These anecdotes present a broad spectrum of attitudes towards Jews and Jewish psychoanalysts. Within them are expressed intensely held transferential feelings which are capable of evoking intense countertransference responses. Let us examine these anecdotes in context, to more fully appreciate their implications.

The first example (1) is intriguing in the patient's expectations that the Jewish psychoanalyst live up to being a member of the People of the Book. The patient is confused by her psychoanalyst's lack of religious commitment. Her confusion was exacerbated by her own need to experience the psychoanalyst as being without the ambivalence and passivity that she experienced in her husband, an ambivalence and passivity that had outraged her own dependency strivings and facilitated her entry into psychoanalysis. *This incident highlights the reality that even when the psychoanalyst attempts to be religiously neutral, neutrality remains difficult to achieve and is still subject to interpretation and transferential distortion.* Indeed, it may be that rigid adherence to this neutrality and to preservation at almost all costs of the therapist's religious anonymity is partly responsible for the reported absence of anti-Semitism as an aspect of the negative transference that so often emerges in treatment, which is, after all, so present in the real world outside of the psychoanalyst's office.

The second vignette (2) reflects the manifold complexities which surround the issue of payment and how these become further intertwined with ancient religious and racial stereotypes. The patient's resentment for rescheduling a session expresses itself in his anger at previously paying for a missed session (albeit with some reason since the second session was at a slightly less convenient time than the first). Nonetheless, the defensive stance which he adopted to voice his objection appeared to arise less from experiences typical of the course of psychoanalysis than from his particular resentment towards a Jewish analyst who would both demand payment and reschedule a session to meet his own religious needs. I noted above that an intense father transference had appeared during the course of a psychoanalysis which the patient, who was actively homosexual, had entered to explore heterosexual options. While ostensibly he was protesting payment, the presence of a stereotype is much more obvious. His comment and further associations revealed that the analyst was no longer experienced as a professional expecting payment, but rather as a usurer demanding excess interest. This interaction over financial matters allowed the patient to explore his general passivity within exploitative situations. He had projected onto Jews the characteristics of being competitive, with a concomittant concern over financial integrity and, ultimately, control over their individual sexual expression. As he explored his competitive feelings toward the analyst, he became more comfortable with experiencing the desire to control his sexuality in nonexploitative circumstances.

In the preceding illustration the superficial issue is the patient's projection that the psychoanalyst was involved in an exploitative process, victimizing the patient financially. While this issue was explored as a resistance — as the patient's problem — the very intensity of his feelings did evoke countertransference. Indeed, in this case the psychoanalyst had been overly flexible regarding payment. His flexibility, in this regard, may reflect his own ambivalence towards this species of libel and his own desire to prove to the patient that he did not conform to this stereotype. Thus, the psychoanalyst is not immune to the influence of stereotypes about his group of origin and belief. It may be that the patient unerringly recognized the therapist's ambivalence and chose appropriately enough to hang him by his own need to placate. However, when the analyst did not flinch from confronting the patient with his use of stereotypes, the patient was ultimately able to explore his competitive and passive behavior expressed with figures toward whom he had experienced anger — an anger that now he had displaced onto the analyst through the vehicle of racial and ethnic stereotypes.

Countertransference issues of greater intensity are presented in the last two vignettes. In the third vignette (3), a group member made an extraordinarily provocative statement. This statement during the course of a group session evoked extreme and not inappropriate anger from the Jewish group members. And as the author has noted elsewhere, the use of ethnic and religious slurs demands that the group leader make an unusual effort to retain his objectivity within the group setting (Halperin, 1981). Indeed, the group leader, himself, was hard pressed to retain the group member in the face of the appropriate rage her remark had provoked among the group members. His countertransference was intense. Moreover, the group setting seemed to demand some instantaneous response and to preclude an exploration of the member's underlying motivation.

At this time, the group leader remembered that the patient in question was a professional who had worked for many years for a Jewish institution and that she had recently returned from her third visit to Israel. It was thus difficult to understand her statement as a product of unalloyed anti-Semitism. The object of the patient's initial attack was an older woman who used both her status as a Holocaust survivor and her interactional style to obsessively control the group interaction. Her control had rarely been challenged and indeed appeared impervious to attack as she prevented the discussion of many issues within the group through her pervasive use of intellectual defense and denial. In this perspective, much of the group's anger towards the "anti-Semitic" member was to a large degree a displacement of its own rage towards the "victim." The dilemma was dealt with by encouraging the offending member to explore her use of racial epithets as a means of expressing anger, but in a manner which ensured that all the group anger would then be displaced onto her. Both the group and the individual then began to deal more realistically and appropriately with their feelings. Indeed, for the other group members, the incident was particularly useful in forcing them to confront their own stereotype of the omnipotent anti-Semite who can only be evaded but never successfully confronted.

This incident evoked an intense countertransference reaction. As the patient was in conjoint treatment, the additional possibility that the anti-Semitic remark directed towards a fellow group member was a displacement of the anger felt towards trhe therapist was explored primarily in her individual treatment. The patient had many borderline features which both encouraged fusion with significant male figures and prevented the formation of any stable relationship with them. Indeed, the course of the patient's treatment had been characterized by constant threats on her part to withdraw from treatment and the fear that the therapist would unilaterally terminate with her. Her anti-Semitic remark was in the service of her resistance to therapy and part and parcel of the process that had prevented her from forming stable male relationships (including with the therapist). Comparably, her frequent visits to Israel and her working for Jewish institutions may be considered a reaction-formation or as evidence of the process of idealization and mirroring which always co-exists with the potential expression of denigrating rage. This has been noted as an aspect of anti-Semitism (Ascherson, 1983).

THE CASE OF HEATHER A.

A more subtle problem is presented in the fourth (4) vignette. The patient, Heather A., is a 28 year-old fashion professional whose closest friends and professional colleagues are Jewish. Her rage was precipitated by a sense of alienation and the fantasy that she was being systematically rejected by the members of her summer house who were Jewish. The particular object of her ire was E., "who's my ideal. She's like Zsa Zsa Gabor." Heather A.'s outburst is more understandable when placed in historical context. Heather A. was the oldest child of a large, fanatically Catholic Irish-American family. Her father was inaccessible except when delivering political and anti-Semitic tirades to which the family listened. Her mother presented herself as a pseudo-helpless woman who dutifully gave birth to a large number of children and then left their care to Heather A. Her entry into therapy was precipitated by her ambivalence towards her profession where she would overidentify with her employees and resent their dependency on her and dependency on men. She would form relationships with inaccessible men and then resent their distance and yet be unable to separate from these idealized figures after the termination of the relationship.

Heather's anti-Semitic outbursts reflect a complex of factors. Of primary importance is her identification with a rabidly anti-Semitic father. Her father became relatively accessible when she listened to his tirades, and his own sense of competence and achievement which would spill over to Heather on such occasions contrasted favorably with her mother's pseudo-helplessness. In this context, her relationship with the psychoanalyst was marked by idealization and mirroring ("I'll never be as good a person as you are") and rage at his being married, inaccessible during vacations, etc. In the illustration, Jewish women, including the psychoanalyst's wife and children, became the successful competitors for paternal attention — only this time it is the idealized and overvalued Jewish psychoanalyst that is the object of her attention rather than the harsh paternal introject.

Heather's anger towards E., her housemate, was compounded out of her idealization of her anger at her inability to successfully mirror E.'s behavior, and her rage at being deprived by E. of the male nurturance that she sought. Above all, both E. and Sheila were viewed as competent women whose Jewishness allowed them to accept their femininity without discarding their autonomy—a feat beyond Heather's mother's pseudo-helplessness. Ultimately, as Heather began to explore her idealization of Jews, she was able to accept her own limitations and was less driven to resort to contempt and denigration as a means of preserving her sense of self and her professional competency.

The process of idealizing the Jewish analyst and its concomitant mirroring need not always lead to expressions of disillusion and anti-Semitic denigration. The individual's identification with the psychoanalyst may lead to the development of countertransference problems of a more subtle variety, as the following case illustrates.

Henry C., a 40 year-old Irish-American, was seen in psychoanalytically-oriented psychotherapy because of problems of work inhibition and social withdrawal. Despite his obvious competence, he had never been able to hold a job for more than a year. His childhood had been characterized by a conflictual and critical relationship with a stepfather who viewed him as an oedipal rival. Indeed, he had a very close, almost symbiotic relationship with his mother. During the course of treatment, Henry began to date Rosalyn, who was both Jewish and strongly identified herself as being Jewish. His mother began to warn him against the consequences of pursuing this relationship and darkly hinted that his Jewish analyst might not be objective.

It has been the author's experience that not infrequently during the course of treatment, non-Jewish patients may start to date or court Jewish partners (although given the demography of middle class New York this is no longer unexpected). As in Henry's case, the non-Jewish patient may start to idealize his Jewish partner and the perceived closeness and flexibility of the Jewish family, etc. Alternatively, during the course of the relationship, this original closeness may be perceived as threatening the loss of the individual's identity, a fear that then is expressed in sarcastic remarks about the presumed clannish quality of the Jewish family. Henry's mother felt threatened by the loss of her symbiotic tie to her son and she responded to this threat by focusing on his partner's and analyst's Jewishness. Henry, himself, preferred his partner being Jewish because of his own fantasies that this would increase his ultimate distance from his controlling mother.

In this situation, the Jewish psychoanalyst must be alert to his ambivalence towards his own religious background. Initially, as the nonJewish patient begins to demonstrate idealizing behaviors, the psychoanalyst may be prone to dismiss it out of hand without attempting to objectively evaluate the positive aspects of the new relationship (as in Henry's case, where his partner appeared to be genuinely tolerant and emotionally open). The analyst's zeal to interpret the new relationship primarily as a displacement of feelings from the psychoanalyst onto another nurturing figure who shares his religious identity—which, or course, needs to be explored—may also reflect his ambivalence about his own background in which warmth and the ability to express feelings may be intertwined with less positive qualities such as the need to overprotect. Indeed, as the psychoanalyst helps the patient to explore the new romantic relationship, he may develop a greater appreciation of his own background. Not surprisingly, many interfaith relationships appear to founder over religious issues: i.e., the religion of the children, or under whose auspices the couple will be married, or what degree of religious observance will be allowed in the home. However, it has been the author's experience that these issues are often epiphenomena and that given both parties' willingness to accept intimacy, satisfactory solutions are available which respect the religious identification of all parties concerned.

As Henry and his partner became increasingly fearful of intimacy, these issues seemed to gather in intensity. It was quite dramatic that Henry developed an interest in an attachment to his "roots" as the time approached for full commitment to Rosalyn. His rapprochement with his past involved both an acceptance of the positive aspects of his personal religious identification and an exploration of his religion's as well as his family's ambivalence towards Jews. This ambivalence extended towards both his prospective partner and his psychoanalyst. The potential for a therapeutic impasse was obvious. However, during the course of the analytic work that fol-

lowed, Henry was able to develop an appreciation that this recrudescence of his ambivalence with its anti-Semitic overtones formed a
significant part of his attempt to preserve distance between himself
and his prospective partner, and in a sense represented the last gasp
of his fears of separation from his family and of engulfment by his
partner's family. Moreover, he was able to appreciate the extent to
which his identification with his father had precluded the formation
of a trusting relationship with significant male authority figures. To
date, Henry is happily married.

I have illustrated how the relationship of the psychoanalyst to the
individual patient can receive closer examination particularly with
regards to the context of the ethnic as well as religious differences or
similarities between patient and psychoanalyst that permeate and
over-determine all aspects of the therapeutic encounter. We will now
consider in greater detail an illustration of this sort of examination in
the case of non-Jewish patients and Jewish therapists.

THE ETHNIC INTERFACE:
THE JEWISH-IRISH DIALOGUE AS A
PARADIGM FOR CONFLICT RESOLUTION

The relationship between Jew and non-Jew has been characterized by alternating periods of cooperation, coexistence, and
violence. The emphasis on the dramatic periods of conflict tends to
overshadow the long periods of fruitful, mutual interaction. On the
personal level, this interaction has been charaterized by idealization
and mirroring and on the other hand by anger, denigration, and dis-
tancing. Ths history of the relationship between the Jews and the Irish is not exempt from this ambivalence and volatility, and the
ambivalence present in society extends itself into the therapeutic relationship. This section explores the process by which the individual
experience of a Jewish psychoanalyst and an Irish analysand is per-
meated by and altered by this historical tradition.

On the level of Irish legend, the Celts of Eire were identified with
the ten tribes of Israel. Although Jews were denied permission to re-
side in the pre-Conquest kingdom of Munster, Jewish merchants requested permission to trade. The kings of Ireland shared with the

British monarchy the fantasy of the New Jerusalem and were crowned with consecrated oil. Tara was equated with Torah, and "the harp that once through Tara's halls" was identified with the harp played by red-haired King David. In modern times, Irishmen and Jews have shared both a tradition of oppression and the reality of being oppressed by a common imperialist (hence the cooperation between the Irish Revolutionary Army and the Irgun Z'vai Leumi in the period prior to the creation of Israel—a cooperation embodied in figures such as Paul O'Dwyer and David Briscoe). There is also a history of ambivalence as exemplified by Irish neutrality during World War II, and by the contradictory perceptions of Cromwell (and the Puritan tradition)—to Jews, the heroic figure who allowed their return to England; to the Irish, the arch-villain who sponsored the Drogheda massacres. Thus, it is less surprising that in *Ulysses*, the novel which explores the Irish past and present—whose author, James Joyce, was obsessed by his ambivalence towards his people and homeland—has as its chief protagonist-hero, Leopold Bloom, a member of Dublin's small Jewish community. In contemporary times, the attempt to revive Gaelic as a modern language has drawn inspiration from the successful revival of Hebrew.

The roots of Irish-Jewish antagonism are deep. Ireland was and is a pre-eminently Catholic country of peasants contained within a rigid hierarchy of landowners (formerly Anglo-Irish Protestants) and the Roman Catholic Church. Jews were charaterized as Christ-killers. On a more sophisticated level, they were viewed as arrogant usurers in contrast with the contemplative Irish poet-peasant. The Irish epithet for Jews, "sheeny," literally means "smart," but was utilized to mean devious, cunning, or guileful. It is an epithet that simultaneously expresses idealization and denigration (Archie Bunker hires a "Heb" lawyer). In this context the conflict emerges between the Jewish psychoanalyst who is the product of an intellectually competitive familial environment which contrasts with the egalitarian Irish jibe at the presumptive intellectual overachiever—"Who does he think he is?" On another level, whatever the sexual constraints of the Jewish home environment, Judaism never encouraged celibacy nor is there anything within the Jewish tradition comparable to the Irish Catholic tradition of sexual inhibition. Nor is the ritualized use of alcohol within Jewish tradition comparable to the complex of bonding and socialization which surrounds alcohol in Irish culture. The presence of these widely differing conceptions of the importance of intellectuality, sexuality, and substance use/abuse inevitably create difficulties in the relationship between the Jewish psychoanalyst and the Irish analysand.

These issues are illustrated in the case of Ophelia. Ophelia was a 40 year-old woman of Irish-American antecedents. At the age of 25, she entered a teaching order of nuns. It was a decision which her family initially viewed with considerable skepticism but which they ultimately accepted because Ophelia had always seemed to be more passive and dependent that their other children. Ophelia became a very competent and respected teacher. At the time of her entry into the Order, the Order had been a rather authoritarian environment removed from the affairs of the world except for its primary mission of providing teachers for parochial schools. However, the Order slowly began to change. Inevitably, Ophelia was forced to confront a world she had sought to escape. She resolved her dilemma by leaving the Order and becoming a lay teacher in a parochial school. She was referred for psychotheapy by a family member who had noted her increasing sense of purposelessness, asthenia, and depression.

In one sense, working with Ophelia was comparable to working with any individual who had just left an authoritarian, hierarchical society. Within the Order, her basic psychosocial needs had been met. However, in her psychoanalysis, it was essential that her analyst appreciate that while joining a religious Order might have reflected some of Ophelia's sexual inhibitions and desire to find psychological support, the essence of her decision to join a spiritual Order was an authentic spiritual calling. And while the psychoanalyst with his different religious background might view the patient's path with some skepticism, her initial decision deserved respect. During the course of treatment, the focus of activity centered on Ophelia's need for authority and her fear of either confronting or disagreeing with authority. In actuality, the Order had provided a "holding environment" in which Ophelia had developed a more secure sense of herself. In fact, this important internal change had been a significant factor in her initial decision to leave. Nonetheless, Ophelia continued to view authority in totalistic terms. During the course of psychoanalytically-oriented psychotherapy, we explored Ophelia's tendency to view her school principal with the same reverence she had previously accorded the mother-superior. Also discussed were her fears of living independently without the sheltering arms of a roommate. Eventually, she was able to work in a more independent fashion and independently expand her social sphere. Her depression lifted. Approximately two years after leaving treatment, she wrote to inform the psychoanalyst of her impending marriage. In working with Ophelia, the issue of intense religious commitment was raised in terms of its effect on the patient (and parenthetically on the psychoanalyst). By regarding the individual's use of a spiritual vocation as part of a process of growth, the psychoanalyst was able to avoid relating to the patient in terms of the polarization, splitting, and overidealization that had previously dominated her life.

The relationship between the psychoanalyst's religious identification and the patient's own religion may express itself in the superficially abstract plane of the "conflict" between religion and psychoanalysis. Freud himself was aware that psychoanalysis might be regarded as a Jewish "cult" opposed to Christianity. Thus, it is not surprising that a nonJewish patient might see psychoanalysis as undermining implicitly his own religious identification or, at the very least, view the psychoanalyst as being inherently opposed to the possession or expression of any intense religious commitment. These issues are illustrated in the following case.

THE CASE OF TARA

Tara, an attractive, devout Catholic mental health professional, was referred for psychotherapy because of intense anxiety, depression, and fears that she was no longer able to work effectively. In addition, she had become increasingly aware of her affectionate feelings for a female coworker. The actual referral was precipitated by her exacerbated anxiety during the course of psychotherapy with a female therapist. In the opening session, Tara openly discussed her many concerns that as a result of entering more intense treatment, she might be forced to renounce or lessen her religious commitment.

The psychoanalyst's initial approach was to reassure Tara that although he did not share her particular religious beliefs, he was quite certain that this would not prevent their working together in a cooperative and constructive manner. Nonetheless, this issue continued to present itself during the course of treatment. Two aspects seemed to be particularly significant in this regard. On the one hand, Tara's religious identification was an important part of her sense of self. Her father was born a Lutheran and had converted to Catholicism after his marriage. Her mother was a devout Catholic. Tara's life had been dominated by the death of her mother at an early age. It seemed that her religious concerns were an element of her identification with her lost mother and her desire to maintain her femininity. Moreover, she identified her father's religion of birth with a stern, unemotional stoicism which denied her the right to feel and to express her feelings. In this context, her continued concern over the loss of her religious identification reflected her concerns over her femininity and her fear of dependency on the psychoanalyst. This fear of dependency on the psychoanalyst would return with renewed force whenever Tara would attempt to mobilize herself socially and act in a more autonomous fashion at work. In this regard, it must be noted that the coworker whose friendship she both sought and avoided was a former nun. Her religious concerns deserved respect but were obviously multidetermined (as was her choice of a Jewish psychoanalyst whose being Jewish provided both support and distance).

Tara's preoccupation with the issue of her sexual orientation prevented her from receiving communion or participating in confession because of her fears of moralistic strictures that might accompany this. At this point, her psychoanalyst suggested that she was assuming a uniformity in attitude among priests as she had previously stereotyped the attitudes of psychoanalysts. Tara had assumed that because her psychoanalyst was a Jewish male he could not be empathetic with either her religious concerns or her sexual orientation. Tara explored her primitive and punitive perspective of both religious observance and the practical aspects of psychoanalytic treatment. She saw her faith and her psychoanalysis in the same totalistic, authoritarian terms without any possible flexibility. Issues of payment, the occasional need to take business trips or to change sessions were discussed with Tara in an open and flexible manner which both underlined the seriousness of the psychoanalytic enterprise while preserving it as a cooperative process.

In Tara's initial search for the sacraments of her faith, the priests she encountered indeed appeared to be moralistic and judgmental. She had made no further effort to seek more sympathetic spiritual counsel. In her psychoanalysis, she explored the process of splitting and/or overidealization which had previously led her to assume that the only valid spiritual experience is necessarily the most punitive. She described herself as feeling uncomfortable when she finally discovered a more open and less judgmental religious setting. In this regard, Tara resembled the members of the conservative groups that have arisen in the aftermath of Vatican II (Scavullo, 1983). Tara was not unique in her assumptions that religious faith necessarily reflects the most harsh and punitive aspects of the superego. It is an attitude that is unfortunately all too common among mental health professionals. It is reflected in the difficulties experienced by mental health professionals in distinguishing between religions and cults because of their facile assumptions that both religions and cults share a rigid, authoritarian disdain for the individual (Halperin, 1983).

Eventually, Tara was able to appreciate that her view of the Church mirrored her own punitive superego and that, in reality, within any organization of the breadth and diversity as the Catholic Church there must necessarily be a wide disparity of approaches to human dilemmas. Tara was able to obtain the spiritual succor she sought and subsequently has been able to participate in a wide variety of lay activities within the Catholic Church. During the course of this therapeutic activity, the psychoanalyst's work reflected his own recognition of the importance of the individual's spiritual identity and that whatever the details of their theologies, all of the great religions consensually adhere to a recognition of the importance of the individual. Tara's growth is the reflection of this belief.

THE CASE OF BRIAN K.

In the illustration that follows, the analyst had to adopt a different approach to confront religious issues. This case concerns a patient who was reluctant to recognize the analyst's Jewishness and to discuss his own Catholicism which was of central importance in his life.

Brian K. is a 30 year-old Catholic from a small midwestern town who came to New York to pursue a career in the theatre. His interests had not been encouraged by his family or community, and he had turned bitterly against them all. The one affiliation from childhood which he retained was his religious identification, and he attended Mass weekly. This was also the one area he refused to discuss in his analysis though many of his dreams were set in churches or involved other religious symbols. Brian's refusal was expressed explicitly and firmly; he would not speak about his religious beliefs because "I just don't want to talk about it." He offered no explanation and would not discuss the matter further. The analyst respected the powerful resistance on this topic and decided to not get into a struggle with the patient. The analyst felt hopeful that with the establishment of an effective working alliance Brian would eventually explore this area.

His initial dream consisted of a church, steeple and all, being removed by a derrick from one foundation to another. In the manner of a patient newly involved in his analysis and eager to please the therapist with a dream, Brian expressed confidence that the dream signified his rebuilding his emotional life on more sturdy grounds. The analyst privately wondered how easily such a transplantation would occur given Brian's insistence on keeping his religious beliefs outside of the analysis. This expectation was highlighted eighteen months later when Brian reported the following:

"I dreamed I was enroute to the cathedral when some mean looking men blocked my way. I had to turn into an Episcopalian Church where I felt endangered everywhere I turned. I knew I wanted to pray, but I was prevented by these dangers."

This dream occured at a time that the patient had been exploring positive feelings toward the analyst which had made the patient anxious. It was clear that a negative transference was beginning to emerge in this dream. The analyst was cast as an evil, disruptive force that prevented the patient from obtaining his goals and in whose presence he felt endangered. Taking this as an opportunity to bring into the analysis the long omitted subject of the patient's Catholicism, the analyst inquired whether Brian viewed the analyst as preventing him from coming to terms with and reaching consolation from his religious beliefs. The patient was unresponsive, overlooked this question, and went on to explore other associations to the dream.

In his next dream the patient reported:

> "I was in a large room, kind of like your office but not your office. The room was filled with books from floor to ceiling. A judge outfitted in the English style proceeded to denounce me. I flew into a rage and began throwing books at him."

Brian was at first devoid of any associations. Eventually he said the judge reminded him of the judge in the movie *Ghandi* who admired Ghandi but nevertheless had to condemn him for his beliefs. The analyst associated that the therapist's office filled with books was suggestive of "people of the book," a reference to Judaism. Brian accepted this and went on to deal with his reluctant awareness of his analyst's Jewishness and his fear that the analyst would condemn him for his religious beliefs just as his family and community had condemned his theatrical, literary, and other personal aspirations. He could not bear the thought that his deepest religious beliefs might be devalued, beliefs that had consoled him through many crises. The analyst felt that throwing the books at the judge/analyst might also reveal deeper anti-Semitic feelings derived from his family and community, but these had not yet emerged in the treatment.

By this point in the analysis, the analyst was confronted with a countertransferential problem which necessitated that he proceed with caution. Raised in a largely Jewish community, the analyst had been imbued with an awareness of the prevalence of anti-Semitism in our society and throughout history. Once, when leaving syna-

gogue as a child, the analyst had been taunted by anti-Semitic
youths. A sensitivity on this topic remains which I take pains to
monitor in my dealing with material which seems anti-Semitic to
me. If Brian were alluding to latent or overt anti-Semitic feelings,
the analyst must, of course, help the patient understand their content and origin. But not everything represents anti-Semitism. Anger
and aggression toward the analyst is present in all analyses. Various
aspects of the therapist may be chosen to symbolize the negative
transference. The selection of the analyst's religion cast in pejorative
light may represent a culturally selected stereotype to which the patient has been exposed or may also reveal that the patient has em-
braced such a belief as his own. The analyst therefore made a
decision at this point not to pursue the issue of anti-Semitism. The
analyst did not want to jeopardize the working alliance which had
emerged by suggesting something that was either untrue or which
may have made the patient unduly defensive. It was sufficient that
whereas initially Brian had refused to talk about religious themes, he
was now in his dreams beginning to address the subject. The analyst
knows that significant unconscious material will recur in dreams,
and issues not confronted now can be dealt with at some future time.
The task was to permit Brian to raise these issues at a pace comfortable to him. An important turning point in Brian's analysis occured
a short time following the above session, as evidenced by the following dream.

> "I was an altar boy setting up for the Mass. The altar was hard to
> reach, and I never did get close to the Crucifix. The Mass could
> not begin before I completed my work. I had to stop to assist an
> elderly priest unravel the entangled chains of the censer."

Brian's associations to the dream focussed on its connection to the
theatre. He had recently assisted in the production of a play in an
auditorium of a church, and an actor who had played the part of a
priest was cast as the priest in this dream. He viewed this man as
benevolent and protective. In contrast to many of his earlier dreams,
the symbol of the analyst does not obstruct or oppose but is now a
benign figure cast as a friendly priest. Together, altar boy and
priest — patient and analyst — collaborate on the censer. Brian's belief
was that freeing him from his internal censorship of feelings would

result in achieving his spiritual and emotional goals. This dream was reminiscent of a pivotal dream of a Jewish patient while he was first becoming committed to his analysis, in which the analyst, cast as a rabbi, was escorted by the patient into a restaurant to meet his friends and family. The patient viewed rabbis as honest, compassionate, learned men of great moral integrity. For that patient, the dream signaled the beginning of a working alliance with the analyst being cast as a benign, paternal figure. The analyst similarly regarded Brian's dream as a statement that analyst and patient would be able to work together collaboratively. This was borne out in ensuing weeks during which a positive transference facilitated Brian's ability to focus on developing deeper interpersonal relationships.

THE CASE OF JOHN

A very different experience was had with another patient.

John, a 25 year-old Irish Catholic, came to treatment because of depression and hypochondriasis. He was preoccupied with fear of recurrence of a childhood cardiac disease although his physician assured him he was cured. In addition, his relationships with women had been short lived, and he did not understand why he could not find a satisfying and lasting relationship. He was raised in an Irish working class neighborhood. His education consisted of parochial elementary schools and Jesuit high school. By 18 he became disillusioned with the church and selected a prestigious secular college. His selection of a Jewish analyst appeared to him at first as coincidental. Later it emerged that he idealized Jews who symbolized to him commitment to intellectual excellence. He continued to maintain contact with some of his former Jesuit instructors who shared his scholarly interests, but he rejected the church because it "lied" to him about "truth." He envisioned Jews as not tied to dogma but as open to diverse ideas. He was also aware of his stereotyping in this matter, but the underlying positive feelings were there. Though anti-Semitism abounded in his childhood community, there was no hint of it throughout the analysis. The positive transference was based on a belief that the therapist was truly interested in his ideas (and indeed, in this obsessional patient, the analyst needed to listen to many ideas before he could help the patient to look at his feelings).

As the analysis progressed, John's anger at the Church subsided as he was able to identify and retain certain values and principles though he continued to reject the formal structure and observance of the religion. The analyst did not share John's condemnation of the Church, but maintained instead a nonjudgmental attitude that facilitated the valuing of that which was good in his religious past. He retained a commitment to social justice and began to serve in a high position in an international social agency. He grew in his ability to translate "Christian" ideals to everyday work.

The religious question aside, John presented various issues that the authors have found often in Irish-Catholic patients: guilt about sexuality that had been exacerbated in early parochial school eduation where male and female clergy had emphasized its sinfulness; fears of homosexuality which often seemed the place to turn if heterosexual contact is to be avoided; anxiety over academic excellence for fear of being singled out as pretentious or ambitious. Interestingly, John, as so many of the authors' Irish-Catholic patients, abstained from alcohol. This departure from a significant aspect of Irish culture may be a factor in such patients seeing themselves as different, in their seeking out analytic treatment which is not readily countenanced in their culture, and in seeking out a Jewish analyst.

A moving experience for the analyst occurred when one patient, Darren, wished to impart his own religious beliefs to this therapist. Religion had emerged in therapy initially as something he dismissed; he felt he had inherited it from his parents and as such he felt compelled to reject its formal trappings. He would have glossed over the discussion of religious themes had the therapist not encouraged the exploration of his values and spiritual sentiments. For example, holiday times were often periods of prolonged depression for Darren related to his feeling emotionally abandoned by his family. Yet there were times that the therapist encouraged the exploration of issues of faith and values. Darren's recollection of his childhood faith in a God who would set things right helped sustain him through these depressive bouts. At times, when his adult skepticism challenged such faith, he could draw upon the values of love and giving, and he could make restitution with his children for what he himself had felt bereft as a child. In therapy, Darren had changed from a deeply depressive character to a position where he felt genuinely optimistic and hopeful in his ability to confront life.

During preparation for termination Darren had been discussing with a Jewish friend his belief in an after-life and was astonished to learn that his friend had no concept of an after-life. Analysis of this issue dealt with Darren's concern about life after analysis and his need to console himself and continue his growth after separation from the analysis (experienced as a loss or death). But he also felt sad for the analyst presuming that he, as a Jew, might not experience this powerful belief which had always provided comfort and reassurance. Having felt consoled in his analysis, he wanted to be assured that the analyst, too, was comforted by inner peace. He brought this to his session in a deeply emotional manner, reporting in detail his conversation with his friend and his subsequent associations to the analyst. He reported feeling surprised at the extent of his preoccupation but was puzzled that in treatment he had regained access to spiritual values, and he felt that it was through the analyst that he had achieved this. How could the analyst help him restore his faith and yet, like his firend, not be a man of faith? He solved this question by concluding that the analyst had not imposed a faith or value on him but had helped him discover his own. He, therefore, assumed that the analyst himself possessed deeply held spiritual values that, though perhaps different from his own, served to sustain the analyst. What was especially moving for the analyst was the development in this patient of a capacity for love and empathy absent in his early family life which had been marked by rigid punitiveness and judgmentalness.

The relationship of the Jewish psychoanalyst and the non-Jewish patient is complex. It may suffer the vicissitudes to which any intense relationship is subject. However, in this instance, the resistance which may develop during the course of any analytic work may receive a certain cultural sanction. The Jew is both idealized and denigrated within our society. Thus, as Freud feared that psychoanalysis would be perceived as a particularly Jewish science, the course of analytic work and the realistic constraints under which it must take place are subject to the idealization and the denigration to which Jews are heir. Some transference and countertransference issues that can develop during the course of the relationship between the Jewish psychoanalyst and the Irish patient have been examined and some approaches are suggested.

REFERENCES

Ascherson, N. Klaus Barbie. *New York Review of Books*, 1983, *30*, 34-36.

Bettelheim, B. Scandal in the family. *New York Review of Books*, 1983, *26*, 36-44.

Bloom, H. Jewish culture in America: Is it possible? *Judaism*, 1982, *31*, 266-74.

Freud, S. Totem and taboo. *Standard Edition of the Complete Works of Sigmund Freud, Vol. 13*. London: Hogarth, 1931.

Goldensohn, S. Psychotherapy for the economically disadvantaged: Contributions from the social sciences. *Journal of the American Academy of Psychoanalysis*, 1981, *9*, 291-303.

Halperin, D. Introduction. In D. Halperin (ed.), *Psychodynamic Perspectives on Religion, Sect, and Cult*. Littleton, Mass: John Wright-PSG, 1983.

Halperin, D. Issues on the supervision of group psychotherapy: Countertransference and the group supervisor's agenda. *Group*, 1981, *5*, 24-32.

Joyce, J. *Ulysses*. New York: Random House, 1932.

Lester, E. Eroticized transference possible in any analytic relationship (Margaret Markham). *Psychiatric News*, May 6, 1983, 36-39.

Scavullo, F. Leonard Feeney: The priest who was more Catholic than the Pope. In D. Halperin (ed.), *Psychodynamic Perspectives on Religion, Sect, and Cult*. Littleton, Mass.: John Wright-PSG, 1983.

Teichner, V., Cadden, J. & Berry, C. The Puerto Rican patient: Some historical, cultural and psychological aspects. *Journal of the American Academy of Psychoanalysis*, 1981, *9*, 277-291.

Section Four
CASE STUDIES IN PSYCHOTHERAPY

Chapter 6

CLINICAL MANIFESTATIONS OF RELIGIOUS CONFLICT IN PSYCHOTHERAPY

PAUL R. BINDLER, Ph.D.

A S a psychotherapist working in an orthodox Jewish community, I have found that many of my religious patients experience conflicts concerning religious practice and conviction in addition to their psychosocial conflicts. Typically, they are extremely concerned about the areas of religious conflict and are anxious to discuss them, either from the outset or as such issues emerge in the course of therapy. Generally, these patients have avoided discussing religious issues with either family members or rabbis because of shame, guilt and embarrassment, or fear of some fantasied reprisal or rejection. Inevitably, they turn to the psychotherapist, often as a last resort, to help them work through these difficulties.

Religious patients often express a preference to work with a religious therapist out of concern that a nonreligious therapist will either not understand them or will attempt to dissuade them from their religious beliefs (Wikler, 1983). This motivation overrides their concerns about discussing "personal matters," such as sex or anger toward a parent, with another religious person who happens to be a psychotherapist.

RELIGIOUS IDENTITY AS A CLINICAL PROBLEM: TRANSFERENCE AND COUNTERTRANSFERENCE

Beginning with the initial interview, religious patients express a variety of responses to my religiousness. Characteristically, there seems to be a feeling of rapport based on ethnic similarities as evidenced, for example, by the usage of Hebrew or Yiddish. My own orthodoxy tends to ease some of the tension and apprehension about entering into therapy, which for some members of the orthodox Jewish community is often an alien and threatening process. On the other hand, some patients are wary of my particular form of orthodoxy and often want to avoid reference to religion because they feel I will disagree with their specific point of view. Such attitudes often betray a particular defensive style and may represent an unconscious attempt to alert me to areas which are taboo and threatening. The avoidance of these issues is rationalized in the guise of religious dissimilarities.

The religious identity of the patient often raises special issues in the course of treatment. These include psychodynamic considerations such as expressions of resistance to treatment, types of conflict, and countertransference responses (Lovinger, 1979; Peteet, 1981; Spero, 1980a, 1981). When the patient expresses a certain value or belief, he may seek confirmation or assurance that he will not be rejected (Beit-Hallahmi, 1975). In particular, he may be seeking help in clarifying conflicting and confusing feelings toward religious observance. Psychotherapists generally have been reluctant to direct their skill to issues that on the surface appear to be conflicts of value and faith rather than neurotic conflicts (Greenacre, 1954; c.f., Bergin, 1980). However, many therapists recognize that maintaining therapeutic neutrality is problematic in such instances, insofar as the therapist's countertransference enters into the therapeutic relationship (Singer, 1977) and his or her attitudes toward religiosity are likely to enter into countertransferential reactions (Lovinger, 1979; Spero, 1981).

The involvement of the therapist in the domain of the patient's religious life should not be allowed to become an added burden to the patient's already taxed ability to cope with the pressures impinging on him, stemming from his guilt and shame. It is inevitable that the patient responds along the religious dimension to the therapist in a manner which corresponds to other significant figures in his or her life. When a patient has a strong sense of urgency to discuss religious difficulties, he often experiences a sense of shame and guilt about revealing the level of his practice and observance to me as another orthodox Jew. While in the initial stages of therapy he may have believed it would be easier talking to me as a therapist, inevitably my own religious background infuses the transference dynamic. Transference fantasies among my patients have included, for example, seeing me as overly righteous and pious.

The therapist who shares the religious beliefs of the patient, or who maintains a positive attitude toward religion, may also develop distortive countertransference responses which can result in therapeutic misalliance (Giovacchini, 1975). The range of negative countertransference reactions includes: (1) "rescue fantasies" to prevent the patient's religious decline; (2) guilt and confusion over values and beliefs triggered by the patient's difficulties manifested in and outside of the transference; (3) negative reactions to subtle idiosyncratic and conflicting differences between patient and therapist; and (4) feelings of inadequacy and insecurity over helping the patient with issues of faith (Lovinger, 1979; Spero, 1981). Concerns of the therapist about the patient's religious doubts may result in distortions in the therapeutic alliance which may be countertherapeutic (Spero, 1981; see also Kahn, 1984). As Spero (1980b) notes, "If we are to be most useful to the [religious patient] who comes for psychotherapy or psychological counseling, we must resist the temptation to blur the distinctions and boundaries between psychotherapy, counseling, religious counseling, social work, and so forth" (p. 181). In helping patients work through religious difficulties, the most fruitful vehicle is to stay within the clinical material as it manifests itself in the religious conflict. To insure that the therapeutic focus is maintained, the therapist must critically monitor his or her own attitudes, values, and emotional responses to the religious needs of the patient (Spero, 1981).

Religious conflicts may be successfully resolved in therapy, depending on a host of variables not the least of which is the therapist's sensitivity to and knowledge of the patient's religious perspectives. When the religious conflict is maintained in the therapeutic focus, characteristic forms of resistance emerge (Peteet, 1981). The patient's religious questions and difficulties may serve to avoid discussion of deeper conflict and to ward off intense anxiety and pain through focusing on less noxious areas of conflict. Typically, such concerns have embedded within them not only a request for "legalistic" or spiritual counselling but also constitute an appeal to the therapist to make a decision, particularly a moral decision, for the patient. According to Peteet (1981), "failure to distinguish among 'religious' resistances to treatment may unnecessarily heighten the patient's sense of conflict between his religious and emotional life, creating an additional iatrogenic resistance" (p. 560).

DIFFERENTIATING HEALTHY AND NEUROTIC RELIGIOSITY

When a patient is plagued by a religious or moral conflict, some clinicians infer that this is a manifestation of some more fundamental neurotic conflict (Pruyser, 1977). This point of view has credence on the assumption that religious conflict is but a manifestation of other psychodynamic issues. And it is surely the case that psychodynamics underwrite all aspects of human expression. However, the clinician must be cautious in asserting that the determinants of psychoneurotic conflict are necessarily to be found in the patient's religious value system. The inclination to make such assertions may increase when patients raise issues of faith in psychotherapy. Certainly a patient's unconscious may exploit his or her religious beliefs as a means of expressing conflict, but this does not identify the religious values *per se* as the neurotogenic agent. Indeed, several theoreticians view religious values and morals as growth-enhancing variables which can promote a sense of well-being and mental health (Bergin, 1980; Bindler and Hankoff, 1980). In Judaism, the emphasis on family cohesiveness, regard for others, and inner moral and spiritual development all have positive influences on the development of personality structure.

In treating the religious patient, one must have a sound basis for differentiating true religiosity from neurotic functioning (Spero, 1980b). In addition, one must carefully consider appropriating a causal role to religious values as the root causes of the pathology. A given belief may not be a causative agent but rather may dynamically reflect ontogenetically primitive ego conflicts. The therapist must assess the current status of the belief system within the entirety of the patient's ego structure. As Spero (1980b) notes, "elements of religion are neurotic only to the degree that such disorder is characteristic of total functioning, predominates, or is autonomous of more mature elements" (p. 155). To abstract the religious element as the source of pathology may devalue its overall contribution to personality. To foster its abandonment may induce disturbances which fracture the psychic structure, especially when the patient, even though in conflict, desires to reestablish an equilibrium within a normative communal belief system.

Of course, the therapist's own religious value and moral posture influences his or her ability to draw this distinction correctly (Apolito, 1970). If the clinician's position is substantially different than the patient's, the therapist may not understand fully the patient's dynamics, and as the evidence suggests, he or she may be more likely to see pathology in values and norms which are quite acceptable and desirable from the standpoint of the patient's cultural milieu. For the patient, the religious system may be appropriate and meaningful in terms of maintaining the overall integrity of the psychic system (Bindler and Hankoff, 1980). If a therapist subscribes to a value system at variance with that of the patient, as a study by Henry, Sims and Spray (1971) suggests is the case in America, and has a negative bias toward religion, there may be unconscious effort on the part of the therapist either to neglect the religious values of the patient, not understand them, or ascribe to them a neurotogenic role. Thus, the patient may be insidiously compelled to abandon his or her religious beliefs.

Spero (1981) recommends the necessity for therapists to distinguish "mature from immature or neurotogenic religious belief" (p. 572) in terms of the belief's adaptiveness and freedom from conflict. Furthermore, a patient's self-examination of religious commitment need not automatically be ascribed to neurotic origins. In many instances, the appropriate vehicle for the resolution of such doubts may be a religious practitioner, typically a rabbi for the population of present concern. Consultation with a rabbi may be sufficient to help the patient, although the effectiveness of such consultations is predicated on the patient's emotional readiness for them which can be facilitated by therapy. In addition, the therapist can help the patient explore why he or she has not discussed these issues with others or, if they have been discussed, the meaning of the response for the patient.

While at times the therapist may find it appropriate to suggest to the patient that he or she consult a religious practitioner for clarification of religious doubts, such recommendations need to be handled cautiously both from the perspective of creating splits in the transference as well as possible countertransferential reactions. Often such recommendations may be motivated by professional reluctance to determine specifically religious or value-laden issues, on the one hand, and obligations on the part of the religious clinician to see that the patient retains a spiritual commitment. These problems may be exaggerated when the patient possesses a religious background, level of intensity of belief, or outlook different than that of the clinician.

Practical realities suggest, however, that many patients are reluctant to seek advice of a rabbi in order to receive help with religious problems. They are often embarrassed and ashamed of their feelings and do not want to present these to the rabbi for fear of rejection or disapproval. They maintain a facade to which they desperately cling. These patients often experience the burden of their problem to such a degree that they feel hopeless and will not be able to change. Since the rabbi represents the exemplar of the community these patients are unwilling to lower their facade in his presence. But they may be willing to discuss these problems with a clinician who represents an outsider, a truly unimpeachable confidant whose religious identity they may feel more capable of ignoring or at least wish to in the initial stages of therapy.

Typically, the patients I have seen who present with problems of faith do reflect psychological conflict in their religious attitudes, feelings, and practice. In these situations, due consideration of religious issues may expose additional clinical material which facilitates clarifying intrapsychic conflict. Yet, outside of a full therapeutic focus, this would not necessarily provide the patient with a vehicle for working through the religious conflict in a systematic fashion. In general, the question for me has been to what extent to focus on religious conflict and work it through in the context of therapy.

The manner in which the patient approaches the conflict will reveal the underlying psychodynamic which defers a more mature religiosity. Generally, the patient's religious issues, embedded in a cluster of neurotic conflict, are a vehicle to express these conflicts and are often a form of acting out, particularly in relation to parental figures, either real or introjects (Lorand, 1962). Lingering infantile response patterns held in check by psychic conflict may provoke crises in faith. For example, the relationship which the patient establishes with God often shares the same dynamic expression and unconscious conflict formation established with father (Rizzuto, 1974). Of primary importance in treatment, therefore, is the manner in which the patient portrays infantile response patterns in the transference.

In assessing underlying neurotogenic forces the therapist must determine the form and emphasis with which the patient's religious beliefs color and modulate the nature of conflicts, compromise formulations, and defensive style. This may be illustrated by the manner in which guilt is experienced and expressed or by the conflicts between personal autonomy and fidelity, brotherhood, and parental authority. The patient's religious concerns not only transfigure neurotic patterns of behavior but also reveal a tension within his incorporation of the religious system's ethos of brotherly love, respect for parents, and so forth (see Blidstein, 1975). The patient's characteristic style of coping with guilt and with object relations reflects the internalization of these values and their relationship with basic ego conflicts. The appropriateness of certain feelings (e.g., guilt) must be assessed in the context of the patient's religious belief system to determine when they have trespassed beyond the limits imposed by the religion into the realms of pathological behavior or thought.

I wish to add at this point that I do not minimize the patient's existential concerns which may be involved in his or her religious difficulties. These may be very real and ultimately need to be attended to in the context of or outside the therapeutic situation (Frankl, 1963). However, seeking the significance and meaning of an individual's religious acts is contingent on the degree of ego maturity achieved. When basic instinctual needs still present themselves as foci for neurotic conflict then the strictures of religious life may be readily incorporated into a harsh superego dynamic which may turn the patient from religion. *In the absence of a reciprocal dynamic between the demands of religious life and the integrity of the self, religious values may become distorted into neurotogenic agents.* In the mature religious personality, an equilibrium is achieved between the need for instinctual gratification and its regulation by religious law. In the immature personality, religious strictures are improperly attuned to the ego's dynamic, fostering regressive modes of behavior. As the ego matures, the demands of religious life can be seen not only as discipline but also as devotion, elevating the spirit and infusing life with meaning.

CASE: JOAN

Joan is a 25 year-old, married, orthodox Jewish woman. When she entered therapy she had been married for $1\frac{1}{2}$ years and had one son. She completed college prior to marriage and worked part-time as a saleswoman until her marriage. She had difficulty taking care of the house, particularly after the birth of her son. She became increasingly anxious and began quarreling frequently with her husband. She was referred to me by a rabbi to whom she and her husband had spoken about some of their problems.

During our early sessions, Joan was guarded and suspicious, in addition to being anxious, and was reluctant to speak freely. She often reported not knowing what to say and would typically ask me to lead her with questions. She was distrustful of me both as a man ("Men don't understand women. Men don't realize how hard it is to take care of the house.") and as an orthodox Jew ("You probably think I'm not a good Jew because I miss my daily prayers."). She was convinced that I thought her crazy. She often alluded to my religiosity, at times feeling that I could better understand her religious motivations and at other times disliking it, convinced that I was judging her actions from the perspective of my religious values. She did not, however, bring her difficulties of faith into therapy initially.

During the first four months of therapy, Joan spent most of the time reporting what happened in her week, particularly those instances when she was either in a panic or phobic. She often talked about difficulties with her child and the lack of her husband's involvement at home. She spoke very little about the past or about her parents. She occasionally talked about her friends but was very reluctant to do so because of the sanction in Jewish law prohibiting gossip and slander about other people. She interpreted this sanction in a very narrow sense, taking it to mean that she would not be able to talk about anybody else to me, even if she did not mention their names.

This was one of the first religious issues to arise in therapy. She had obviously turned this restriction into a defensive maneuver to avoid confronting her feelings about certain object relations and, more fundamentally, as a defense against hostility and rage. I explained to her that in the context of therapy there was some flexibility in curtailing the limits of this restriction, since talking was part of the cure (based on justifications taught to me by my religious advisors). However, Joan remained reluctant, expressing the fear that if she talked about other people she would be punished by God.

Initially wary of entering into dogmatic debate with her, I encouraged her to talk to a rabbi whom she trusted to help clarify matters. She agreed to do so but then kept putting it off, providing numerous excuses for not talking to the rabbi. This went on for several weeks, at which time I suggested that she was not asking the rabbi perhaps because she suspected that he would agree that she was under no restriction to talk freely in therapy and would no longer have an excuse to avoid expressing her feelings concerning other people. She strenuously objected to this suggestion but thereby also became angry with me for the first time. I inquired about her anger with me. She felt that I did not believe her and that I thought she was lying. I took this opportunity to explain that at times I would point out things like this not because I felt she was lying but because people sometimes unconsciously block true feelings when these feelings provoke a lot of anxiety. We talked about this and she seemed to accept it. She admitted that there might be something to what I said and that she knew at times she had feelings that she did not want to confront, and this may have been one of those times. Later that week she talked to a rabbi and was indeed assured that she could express herself more freely in therapy.

The approval by the rabbi of my interpretation allowed Joan to be more open about her feelings. She began to express her feeling that many of her friends were insincere in their religious beliefs and were not adequately devoted to their prayers and ritual practice. She thought they were hypocrites, often doing things not in accordance with the spirit, if not the practice of Jewish law. I asked what particularly bothered her about this. She reported feeling that people often were too liberal in talking "badly" about other people, that they were "slanderous" and "insulting." She also felt guilty when she listened to her friends talking this way, which furthered her avoiding other people. Joan seemed essentially to be talking about herself. Talking about her projected perceptions of others was at this point less threatening for her than talking directly about her own religious practice.

Joan had also been very reluctant to talk about her feelings toward her parents. She told me that "all therapists want to blame everything on the parents" and that she was afraid I would cause her to hate her parents and turn her against them, even though she loved them very much. This reaction-formed attitude was, in my estimation, very strong at this time and could not be directly interpreted. Instead, I asked her to tell me about her religious upbringing and how her parents viewed religion. She described her father as a very pious and devout person who adhered strictly to Jewish law and who was very intolerant when people did not act accordingly. He also had little tolerance for "those people who emphasized 'spirituality' instead of practice." While her mother did not come from a home as religious as her father's, she nevertheless acquiesced to his perspective and lifestyle.

I asked her how she felt about all this, especially in view of the fact that she had taken on a "spiritual bent." Beginning in high school, Joan had decided to focus her practice on those aspects of Judaism that emphasized spirituality, such as praying, meditating, and reciting the Psalms, rather than studying details of the law. She admitted that she felt her father was "perhaps" a little too harsh in his outlook and that she felt a more evenly-balanced spiritual outlook was important. She would not say more at this time. She felt uncomfortable "criticising" her father's outlook and wanted to stop talking about him. In this session she had in fact become increasingly anxious when talking about her childhood home life.

In the next session she reported feeling guilty about talking the way she had about her friends and parents. She did not want to judge them; it was not her place, but God's. I pointed out that when she talked about these matters she became anxious and felt guilty, which she acknowledged. I then asked her if she had some negative feelings about her own level of practice. She became very angry with me and accused me of thinkinng she was bad and added that even asking her such a thing proved that I must be thinking bad thoughts about her. She wished to talk no more about it and remained angry and annoyed for the remainder of the session. Joan's anger with me, indeed her criticism of me, related to her feeling that it is God who ought to judge other people, not her. However, she felt that I was compelling her to talk and that I, as a therapist, was then judging what she said in response to my "compelling" her to talk.

During the next session, Joan was very apologetic for getting so angry with me. I reassured her that it was all right to feel angry but that it was important to understand why my question in the previous session had provoked in her such a strong reaction. At this point she began to talk about her own religious misgivings. She recently felt very weak in her religious practice. She skipped many of her prayers, something which she had never done in past years. Her religious beliefs were losing their significance and her convictions were weakening. I inquired why she felt this way. She answered that for a long time she thought of the world as a very cruel place; there were always wars, starvation, the Holocaust, and so on. She could not understand why God had created such a terrible world...that He *could* have made a world of peace and contentment but did not.

Joan became increasingly anxious as she talked about this material. I asked her to tell me more about what she was feeling. She said that she was afraid that God would punish her for thinking such terrible thoughts. She had been afraid for a long time that many of the things that were happening in her life were a result of Divine punishment for her "evil thoughts." Further, she was afraid her ambivalent feelings would influence her children; she did not want them to grow up with negative religious attitudes.

I asked Joan if she had ever tried to talk to anybody about these feelings rather than carrying around such an enormous burden all on her own. She said that she had not. She added that she was very ashamed to talk to anyone about these feelings and that I was the first person with whom she had ever been open about them. She then acknowledged that she did not want to continue to feel this way. I asked her if she would be willing to talk about her religious feelings in the course of therapy. Still somewhat reluctant, she agreed. She was sure, though, that talking about these feelings would evoke more of God's wrath. At this point I drew an analogy between psychotherapy and the Jewish process of repentance. I told her we all have unconscious feelings that tend to take us away from our religious convictions and that the Jewish sages understood this problem. I suggested to her that Jewish law encouraged people to explore these unconscious feelings, to bring them into the open and transform them into more positive feelings (for an elaboration of this view, see Bindler, 1984). In therapy she could transform her negative sentiments into more positive and sincere ones. Joan ostensibly accepted this and said she would be willing to try.

In a subsequent session I asked Joan to tell me how long she had felt negatively about religion. She remembered feeling disenchanted even in high school. She thought that Judaism placed too much emphasis on "law" rather than "love." I asked her what her life was like at this time. She told me she was very depressed, had no friends, and spent much of her time reading novels. She felt her life had no purpose or meaning. She became increasingly concerned with the cruelty in the world and the lack of love between people. At about this time in her life she became obsessively preoccupied with the idea that God was constantly watching over her and that her psychological conflicts were punishment for her antireligious thoughts.

I asked her about her relationship with her parents during this period. She no longer resisted my inquiry as much as she had previously done. She told me that her father was constantly upset about her school performance and her lack of outside social interests. He would often lecture her about her problems and demand that she "shape up." He never seemed able to "discuss" these problems with her, and she experienced him as unilaterally concerned with his own opinion. Joan was very hurt by his disappointment, feeling she failed his expectations. Her mother was similarly upset and concerned and would often yell at her for being "such a mess." Joan was very hurt by what she perceived as rejection and lack of support. Upon asking her how she felt about this, she immediately incriminated herself. She said she deserved the way they responded to her, just as she deserved God's punishment, because she was basically no good and did not "deserve anything but what she got."

At this point, Joan brought up a recurrent dream which she had for some time but had been reluctant to talk about in therapy. In the dream, the world was in the midst of a war. Joan found herself lost, wandering down an empty and desolate road with signs of destruction all around. She said she somehow knew her parents were still alive in this war but did not know where they were. She felt in the dream that she wanted to be with them but was sure they had gone off somewhere, leaving her behind. She felt very alone and scared in the dream, did not know where to go or what to do, and felt that she was going to die. She also experienced herself in the dream as being enraged and angry.

I asked her if she could tell what in the dream made her so angry. She replied that she always assumed that it was her anger at God for allowing this terrible destruction to occur and added that earlier she had found it difficult to bring up the dream because she was ashamed at having these feelings about God. I interpreted her feeling abandoned by her parents as another source of anger, that she felt rejected by them and that they did not care for her. I also pointed out that she felt abandoned and rejected by God in the same way she felt abandoned by her parents, and her perception of God's cruelty was similar to her perception of her father's harshness and aloofness. At this point Joan began to cry profusely. She also became very angry but now expressed this anger not at me but at her father. She acknowledged the meaningfulness of my interpretation and blurted out, now with intense feeling, that she felt there was never anything she could do to please her father, that he never complimented her, that she was never good enough. She always felt guilty and ashamed that she could never do anything right in his eyes, feelings which were reinforced by her father's constantly accusing her of never being diligent enough in her religious practice. Her religious beliefs were always a source of torment to her, a standard she could never fulfill, and so she derived no comfort from religion.

Joan desperately sought closeness with and attention from her father but was never successful. As she became older, she began to feel that the source of her misery was God because of her failures as a daughter, but also because of her failures as an orthodox woman. She began to transfer to God her rage toward her father. She could not tolerate the enormity of the conflict. The rage which she experienced against both her father and God was intolerable. She felt increasingly guilty and ashamed, and so she ultimately suppressed the conflict, reversing and displacing her angry and insincere feelings onto the minutae of her phobic behaviors, in her troublesome dreams, and in obsessive thoughts about the "general cruelty" in the world. Joan preserved her defenses by rationalizing her feelings as an objective assessment of the world. She admitted to me that one of the difficulties in talking about these feelings was her thought that I would simply disagree with her and think her both "unreligious and crazy." She felt I would be as deceived as other religious people in ignoring the reality of the world. She thought I might have repressed my own genuine feelings and rationalized how God and such cruelty could co-exist. This world view served initially as a compromise formulation, allowing some of her anger to emerge without letting out the enormity of her rage, particularly against her father.

By the end of the first year, Joan slowly had begun to fill in the gaps about her past and her relationship with her parents. The emotional catharsis she had achieved gradually enabled her to explore the bottled up feelings of anger of which she had been so scared. We also continued to talk about religious feelings. As she explored more openly and confronted her feelings toward her parents and their religious world, she began to see that she was not inextricably bound to their thinking and perceptions and that her own religious needs and views were also legitimate from the standpoint of orthodox Judaism. She started to pray more regularly and no longer found ritual observance burdensome. Within a year and a half into therapy, she came to enjoy more fully the religious aspects of her life and found that they gave her existence new meaning and hope.

Joan also began to see her parents in a new way. She no longer experienced their behavior as malicious but understood they had done the best they could in raising her. This altered perception allowed her to feel that she could more sincerely obey the commandment to honor one's parents without the guilt and negative feelings she previously experienced. In confronting her feelings toward her parents, her guilt and shame, and in validating her own viewpoints about religion and the world, Joan experienced an increase in her self-worth and self-esteem.

Joan's response to and experience of God was clearly influenced by the manner in which her father viewed God and the vacuousness she experienced in his approach and by her personal feelings toward her father. I believe that via therapy the insights Joan gained into her transference feelings were helpful both for her religious difficulties and for her object relations. In reviewing my method in this case, it seems that the first significant step in therapy was enabling Joan to experience and acknowledge her anger toward me. In the initial phases of the work, the therapeutic situation constituted a satisfactory "holding environment" in which some of Joan's aggression and rage could be experienced without the reprisals she anticipated. This allowed Joan to develop trust in me and eased the expectation that I, as an orthodox male, would inevitably be punitive in the way she experienced her father and God. That she could come to terms with some of her feelings toward me as a male and as a co-religionist provided the initial opening for further exploration of her feelings toward her father and God.

DISCUSSION

The case presented here illustrates the working through of basic
psychological conflicts in religious patients as an important element
in the resolution of religious conflicts and vice-versa. With the resolution of religious and psychosocial conflict in tandem, these individuals feel better, more hopeful, and more free to pursue the kind of
life they want.

From the standpoint of technique, the therapist must differentiate conflict and pathology from appropriate religious practice. This
discernment presumes that the therapist has or can acquire sufficient
familiarity with the patient's religious system. In areas of religious
conflict, the therapist's main task is to focus on the psychodynamic
conflicts which underly issues of faith. Typically, issues of religious
doubt reflect regressions to more infantile modes of behavior and
thought in which one's relationship with God is restricted by negative object relations established with parents. The alleviation of religious conflict is often facilitated by working through the major
intrapsychic conflicts and the factors contributing to poor object relations.

The success of this venture is also predicated on the therapist's
successful management of transference and countertransference. On
the one hand, the therapist must allow the patient freely to express
feelings toward the therapist which are founded on parental and religious imagos. The transference becomes the vehicle in which the patient can clarify and confront repressed feelings which inhibit a more
mature religious identity. On the other hand, the therapist's response
will be determined in part by his or her knowledge, sensitivity, and
attitudes toward the patient's religious beliefs. Both negative and
positive feelings on the part of the therapist may obstruct therapeutic
progress and the resolution of religious issues. Therapists with negative religious attitudes, on the one hand, may foster the abandonment of religious beliefs on the part of the patient, which is ethically
objectionable as well as clinically problematic. On the other hand,
the therapist who has positive feelings may manifest certain countertransference responses which reduce his or her function as a clinician (Spero, 1980a, 1981).

I clearly have assumed that therapists' values and religious attitudes influence their work in psychotherapy and that conflicts of value enter into the work of all therapy (Bindler and Hankoff, 1980). In the work I presented, I shared the same basic religious system as the patient and therefore felt comfortable and knowledgeable enough to maintain a therapeutic focus on conflicts of faith. I tried primarily to center the work on clarifying and working through the underlying neurotic basis of the conflict so as to allow the patient to re-establish a more mature encounter with religion.

Sharing the patient's belief system can provide a mutual background from which to work, allowing the therapist to more accurately interpret and distinguish pathology from culturally acceptable modes of behavior that may seem alien to a therapist of another orientation (e.g., Karno and Morales, 1971). With orthodox Jewish patients, while they may employ certain aspects of religious law defensively, there is a body of law that must be respected. Patients certainly do use religious laws defensively, justifying their lack of expression of feelings by appealing to these laws. While this must be interpreted to the patient, the therapist at the same time must respect the patient's adherence to the laws. The clinician should know when and how these laws do apply and when they are not applicable to psychotherapy (e.g., Kahn, 1984). Consulting when necessary with an appropriate religious practitioner (e.g., a rabbi) for information concerning obligations and practice is helpful in reaching such understanding. In the case reported in the present chapter there were, at times, issues relating to Jewish law as it pertained to the work in therapy. When such issues arose, I consulted with a rabbi to determine what the law required in the particular case in terms of what was permitted and prohibited.

Recent developments in the areas of ethno-psychology and psychiatry represent one response to the demand that therapists be more sensitive to the religious, ethnic, and cultural requirements of the patients they serve (McGoldrick, Pearce, and Giordano, 1982). In this spirit, therapists must attune themselves to the specific needs and requirements of the religious patient in order to ensure adequate and ethical treatment. To ignore these demands or to uncritically attribute pathology to religious beliefs is to ignore the potential of the patient's religion to stimulate psychological maturity, to infuse life with meaning, and to enhance spiritual fulfillment.

REFERENCES

Apolito, A. Psychoanalysis and religion. *American Journal of Psychoanalysis*, 1970, *30*, 115-126.

Beit-Hallahmi, B. Encountering orthodox religion in psychotherapy. *Psychotherapy: Theory, Research and Practice*, 1975, *12*, 357-359.

Bergin, A.E. Psychotherapy and religious values. *Journal of Consulting and Clinical Psychology*, 1980, *48*, 95-105.

Bindler, P.R. Self-awareness (*cheshbon hanefesh*) and self-analysis. In P. Kahn (ed.), *Proceedings of the Association of Orthodox Jewish Scientists*, 1984, *7*, 123-152.

Bindler, P.R. & Hankoff, L.D. *Jewish law and psychotherapeutic values*. Paper presented at the eighty-eighth annual convention of the American Psychological Association, Montreal, Canada, September 1980.

Blidstein, G. *Honor Thy Father and Mother*. New York: Ktav, 1975.

Frankl, V.E. *Man's Search for Meaning: An Introduction to Logotherapy*. New York: Simon and Shuster, 1963.

Giovacchini, P. *Tactics and Techniques of Psychoanalytic Therapy*. New York: Aronson, 1975.

Greenacre, P. The role of transference. *Journal of the American Psychoanalytic Association*, 1954, *2*, 671-684.

Henry, W.E., Sims, J.H. & Spray, S.L. *The Fifth Profession: Becoming a Psychotherapist*. San Francisco: Jossey-Bass, 1971.

Kahn, P. Psychotherapy and the commandment to reprove. In P. Kahn (ed.), *Proceedings of the Association of Orthodox Jewish Scientists*, 1984, *7*, 37-49.

Karno, M. & Morales, A. A community mental health service for Mexican-Americans in a metropolis. *Comprehensive Psychiatry*, 1971, *12*, 115-121.

Lorand, S. Psychoanalytic therapy of religious devotees. *International Journal of Psychoanalysis*, 1962, *43*, 50-56.

Lovinger, R.J. Therapeutic strategies with "religious" resistances. *Psychotherapy: Theory, Research and Practice*, 1979, *16*, 419-427.

McGoldrick, M., Pearce, J.K. & Giordano, J. *Ethnicity and Family Therapy*. New York: The Guilford Press, 1982.

Peteet, J.R. Issues in the treatment of religious patients. *American Journal of Psychotherapy*, 1981, *35*, 559-564.

Pruyser, P. The seamy side of current religious belief. *Bulletin of the Menninger Clinic*, 1977, *41*, 329-348.

Rizzuto, A.M. Object relations and the formation of the image of God. *British Journal of Medical Psychology*, 1974, *47*, 83-99.

Singer, E. The fiction of analytic anonymity. In K. Frank (ed.), *The Human Dimension in Psychoanalytic Practice*. New York: Grune and Stratton, 1977.

Spero, M.H. The contemporary penitent personality: Diagnostic, treatment, and ethical considerations with a particular type of religious patient. *Journal of Psychology and Judaism*, 1980a, *4*, 133-191.

Spero, M.H. Countertransference in religious therapists of religious patients. *American Journal of Psychotherapy*, 1981, *35*, 565-578.

Spero, M.H. *Judaism and Psychology: Halakhic Perspectives*. New York: Ktav, 1980b.

Wikler, M.E. *The meaning of the therapist's religious identity to orthodox Jewish clients*. Unpublished doctoral dissertation, Yeshiva University, New York, 1983.

Chapter 7

THE REDISCOVERY OF SPIRITUALITY THROUGH PSYCHOTHERAPY

SEYMOUR W. APPLEBAUM, M.D.

AN increasingly holistic perspective in psychiatry and psychotherapy has developed over the past decades, starting with an appreciation of the interaction between mind and body and expanding more recently to include the spiritual. The spiritual/religious dimension of the human personality is a vital component in human health. My use of the concept of spirituality in psychotherapy, as well as a definition of that term for the purpose of this paper, is an operational one. I am not attempting to deal with what spirit is in an absolute sense. The reader is welcome to conceptualize what I am saying in naturalistic or transcendent terms and hopefully will find each perspective useful, and maybe ultimately partially true.

DEFINITION OF THE SPIRITUAL DIMENSION

The working definition of spirit that I am using in this paper includes a number of discreet processes that are encountered within the human psyche. I hope to show that treating these processes as a unified entity called "spirit" makes working with these processes in psychotherapy more meaningful and more effective.

For purposes of simplification, the complex realm called "spirit" can be divided into three main categories: the humanistic elements, the mystical/transcendent, and the distinctly religious. The humanistic element is an expression of those aspects that make man a unique being apart from his biological endowment. They include qualities which result from man's development and operating within a culture and society and in the development of personality. I use the term spiritual in relation to those aspects of man's human qualities that move toward development in the highest possible degree. The Human Potential Movement focuses on many areas of this concept. Many of the secular philosophies, systems of ethics, and a general sense of the higher art of living are expansions of man's uniqueness. The spiritual approach postulates that it is possible to go beyond even these boundaries toward further enriched, if not yet fully conceived, states inherent in man's humanity. Obviously the human condition is not always favorable to man's optimum development and functioning and besets man with a host of problems which limit and thwart his development to full potential. A humanistic perspective further postulates that somehow, somewhere, ultimate good will arise from the whole human experience, not only in immediate visible ways but in more subtle or remote ways which we cannot now fathom and which make the whole enterprise worthwhile.

What most people identify as "religious," the second component of spirit, is an organized "God idea" relating to a transcendent being or purpose; a credo, an institution, a community, many communities, generally having historic components, usually founded by enlightened or unique individuals who had some greater sense or access to the ultimate (prophets and teachers) and usually embodied in some written form and expressed in the form of specific rituals. Religion does not have a monopoly on ethical concerns, but it does connect with ethical concerns because ethical concerns are usually a fundamental part of most Eastern and Western religions, and because the religions provide a rationale for ethical behavior and a way of defining that behavior. Aspects of an individual's more or less institutionalized religious forms or beliefs are usually the most directly obvious component of human spirituality but by no means the only significant or even necessary component.

Mystical and transcendent concepts arise within any religion both at its source and ongoing role in history and hopefully in the individual practitioner. All religions, for example, propose a relationship between man with God as His being responsible for existence on earth, and the devotees want to please God and believe in religious tenets. Spiritual belief is thus a channel by which God and the human being can be drawn together.

Mystical, transcendent, and revelatory experiences and an awareness of the presence of God are important parts of any organized religion. What I have seen in my clinical practice and hope to present some sense of in this chapter is that patients in therapy demonstrate authentic mystical and transcendent experiences whether or not defined by themselves or others as traditionally religious.

Consciousness and a sense of being an "I" are essential parts of the experience of being human and can be involved in the mystical component of spirit. The growth of self-awareness, a deepening of this sense of "I," and the development of a mature identity are part of what is necessary in normal human development. There are many times in most persons' lives when some degree of enhancement of this consciousness exists. Sometimes these are called peak experiences, and may sometimes be unpleasant but still ultra-intense and ultra-real to the individual. Disturbances of consciousness and alteration of self and reality boundaries may also occur in pathological states, but these are usually qualitatively recognizable as aberrations of healthier expansions of consciousness. There are other states of consciousness which, on a lesser scale, may exist as intuitions, and on a larger scale, may expand into creativity, and on a still larger scale may become fully mystical and expand into an intimate relationship with nature, the cosmos, and God.

My point is that there is a realm of normal spirit, even if supranormal, which is an expansion of consciousness, encompassing intuition, creativity, and mystical experience. This realm may be extremely health-producing and integrative when brought into a proper relationship with the whole of the psyche. Since these processes exist whether or not we seek them out, and often may exist in less than ideal forms, it becomes the responsibility of the therapist to understand and direct these experiences into the health-producing role which they are meant to have. Furthermore, it may be possible in some cases to evoke these processes, which may be desirable during treatment where they can be guided toward therapeutic results. The goal may be not complete acceptance of institutionalized religious beliefs and practices, but rather a rediscovery of the essential human quality of spirituality, as an end in itself or as prelude to more sustained interest in institutionalized religious expressions.

CASE: MR. M. — REDISCOVERY OF SPIRITUALITY IN A JEWISH PATIENT

I first met Mr. M. in 1981 when he was 24 years old. He was a highly intelligent, articulate, handsome, single, Jewish Caucasian. He had graduated from college just prior to coming to see me. He worked episodically as a night manager in a small hotel owned by a relative. He had moved away from his parents' home shortly after finishing college and was sharing an apartment with two male friends. About half the time he stayed at his girlfriend's apartment. Mr. M. revealed later that he was receiving a subsidy from his parents that made up more than half of his living expenses, though he did not present this issue during the early visit.

The patient first came to see me because of his parents' insistence that he was drifting since his college graduation, and the feeling that there was something psychologically wrong with him, that he would continue to drift and might never get his life together. In addition, they were concerned that he was frequently depressed, sometimes seriously so, for stretches ranging from days to weeks. They viewed his off-and-on relationship with his girlfriend as going nowhere and reflecting the same tendency to drift. Mr. M.'s parents were troubled by his increased irritability with them and felt that they often had to tiptoe around him, particularly his father who was a gentle and tactful individual. His mother was more aggressive and outspoken, and she and Mr. M. would often get into bruising fights. They became increasingly worried after Mr. M. moved out of their home to share an apartment with two young men of whom they did not approve. His parents were fearful that he would start using drugs and drift even deeper into a deviant lifestyle. And, although they did not state this as a reason for asking him to see me, they revealed a good deal of concern about his defection from the family's orthodox Jewish practice a few years earlier. Mr. M.'s parents were both Holocaust survivors and lived through the horrors of a death camp while maintaining not only their lives but also a strong faith in Judaism and God. They were heartbroken that Mr. M. was not following in this path and felt that it was a sign of some illness that was growing in him and disrupting his life.

The parents asked Mr. M. to see me because I am orthodox and felt that perhaps I could help him in a religious as well as a psychological sense. They personally were hesitant to come in, although they were seen from time to time by myself and my wife who is a psychiatric social worker. Yet they studiously avoided becoming involved in any regular family therapy program, despite a number of requests to do so.

Mr. M.'s reasons for coming in were not completely clear for a long time. He initially denied any serious psychological problems and denied even more vehemently that he was drifting. He stated emphatically that having worked very hard in college he felt that he was entitled to a "leave of absence." He had been very close to a strong "A" average in the pre-medical program, but was not sure what he wanted to do with his life. He now wished to take stock of his future direction. Overtly, he wanted me as an ally against his parents. He hoped I would give him a "clean bill of health" to neutralize the harassment he felt from his parents — to help get them off his back. He did not feel helpless about this but felt constrained at how vigorously and harshly he put them in their place, and he admitted to some guilt about the distress they were undergoing because of what he deemed to be a misperception of his current course of action.

By way of additional background on the family, Mr. M. was the middle child of three. A sister six years older lived in Israel, and a sister who was just one year younger lived on her own in an apartment. She had a successful job in a fairly sophisticated industry. She was unmarried, with a boyfriend of five years, and like Mr. M. was unable to make a decision about marriage and commitment. Apparently Mr. M. was the last one to move out of the parents' home.

In the course of one and one-half years of active therapy in which I saw Mr. M. more or less regularly, a number of spiritually related topics emerged. One of these was his relationship to his former orthodox upbringing and yeshiva education with which he broke during his late adolescence. He still wanted to feel as part of the Jewish people and searched for a new and relevant definition of that relationship. He wanted to maintain a cordial relationship with his parents, if they would allow this, but also wanted the right to be radically different than they were in the vital areas of his nonreligiosity and different lifestyle. He wanted to find his own answers to the fundamental questions of life, if he could. This was true in spite of the fact that his break with orthodoxy and his parents involved a loss of belief in God, which was quite unpleasant for him because it meant the loss of faith in the dominance of good in the world. The alternative, with which he grappled painfully, was a universe in which evil was very powerful, sometimes overwhelming, and terrifying for him. He could find some taste of meaningfulness and beauty in what he experienced in nature during his many camping and hiking trips, but saw human civilization as corrupt and hopeless and could not commit himself to being a significant part of this society.

The early phase of therapy involved my attempt to form a therapeutic alliance with him, which was more difficult than usual. M. was very defensive about revealing anything that would seem to justify his parents, critical view of him. He tried to demonstrate his verbal facility, his intelligence, and his sincerity, and to give a strong positive impression of the constructive uses to which he was putting his present time, even though it might seem like drifting to an outsider. He wanted me to know that he read a lot; wrote poetry; spent a lot of time talking to people; and did much serious thinking about himself, about life, and his future, and his place in the broad scheme of things. His holding back on a choice of a career, he re-stated numerous times, was a responsible act because it was important that he use his life wisely and not move in any firm direction until it was clear that it was the correct direction.

When his ambivalent relationship with his girlfriend came up in discussion, he claimed it reflected his unwillingness to become more involved than he genuinely was ready for, or that he thought she was ready for. He felt he loved her and she loved him, but he was distressed by some of her shortcomings. He felt she was quite a dependent person, originally on her parents and now on him and her parents alternately, sometimes to the point of clinging, that she lacked sufficient self-confidence and was at least mildly depressed most of the time. He portrayed his involvement in this relationship as somewhat selfless; that he was interested in her and that because he felt he could be good for her he did not want to break it off, hoping that she would mature and that he could work things out.

Although he originally presented his coming to see me as his parents' idea and suggested that he would have been satisfied with limited goals (primarily getting a clean bill of health from me), his involvement in therapy deepened. A number of factors contributed to the consolidation of our working alliance and the continuity of therapy. One was my genuine affection for him as a person, and another was my admiration for his strengths in spite of his many serious, if not well-confronted, difficulties. I was able to help him verbalize his guilt about the pain his recent years of rebellious behavior were causing his parents, as well as the anger which their criticism caused him.

M. expressed himself in the following way during one early session:

> "I went over to my parents' house and it ended up in a fighting match, especially with my mother. It makes me so mad! I don't go over there so often now, but I know that they feel bad if I don't show up at all, at least sometimes. I always promise myself that somehow I will avoid fighting with them, but it always happens. I guess they can't help giving me digs about the fact that I am still not in school, or that I don't have a regular job, or have a clear direction in life. I guess I get kind of crackly when they raise these issues. My father tries to soften the blow; he is a softer guy. If it was only my mother I think I would never go home again. Sometimes I think I really hate her. I do love my father, and I really can't stand to hurt him. He tries to put on a brave exterior and reason with me. I can talk to him rationally, and he seems to be more understanding, although I know he doesn't really agree.

I wish I could just hate them, period, and never go home. A clean break would be much easier. But I know how much they went through under Hitler, and how hard they struggled to make it in America, and did make it, and how hard they worked to give my sisters and me a good home, a good education, and whatever money could buy. They are not rich, but they have done well, which speaks well of them. They are both very hardworking. They're both good business people; honest, which in *this* society says a lot. I hate business, though — it's too cut-throat, even when you need money, but what's the point? I usually go over there a couple of hours every other week. They keep pushing me to come for Sabbath, but that would be fatal. They and most of their neighbors know I'm not observant anymore, but I know it would hurt them if I drove up or left before the end of Sabbath, and I couldn't stand to spend 24 hours with them. Believe me, Doc, if I spent that much time with them, I'd *really* need you."

I suggested to M. that even if he did not spend with them 24 "deadly hours" of Sabbath, it seemed that *any* time spent with them got on his nerves. His reply was, "That's why I spend so little time with them, as seldom as possible." "But," I replied, "they seem to effect you even when you're not there with them — they seem to be here with us right now. This relationship with your parents has some good *and* bad points." In this and a number of other ways I tried to help M. feel comfortable to discuss his disturbed feelings without feeling that he was a bad person, a failure, or that the harsh tone of his parents' criticism might really be justified, or that he really was something akin to a scoundrel or mental case, or both (which was of course an exaggeration of his parents' view, but not a total misconception of it).

M. responded:

"You know, Doc, I really love my parents — they worked so hard to bring us up. They are sincere, good people. My mother will kill herself to do things for neighbors, and even strangers. She is really very generous — but she certainly is blunt. She has no sensitivity, no understanding of how someone can be different from her, especially her children. I really miss being orthodox. I used to enjoy it. *Shabbas* [Sabbath] was a day of beauty for me. I wish I hadn't lost my religious faith — but it was only a security blanket.

I wish they would understand. I didn't stop being religious *just* so
I could have more fun out of life! The year I spent in Israel when
I was 18, and went to yeshiva, was a very strange year for me. In
some ways I was very homesick, but I felt good to be away from
home. I suddenly felt I didn't need my parents to protect me.
They are loving, but very overprotective. They always think they
know what is best for all of us. My sister moved as far away [to
Israel] as she could. My father used to sit at the window and cry
for a long time after she left. What did *she* do that was so terrible?
They just couldn't let go of her. I can understand that, though,
when I think of how much they lost — their family, friends, their
whole world, their whole life. Dragged away from their homes
when they were teenagers — they never had what I had. All they
had was barbed wire and hunger, and those cold, murderous cat-
tle cars, and hellish gas chambers, and the horrible stench of
death. They survived, by some series of miracles, and to survive
the death camps was no easy job. They never even lost faith!
They even managed to keep some traces of religious practices in
the shadow of that torture and death, under the noses of the Nazis. They managed to encourage and revive other people with
them in the camp, with the hope that God had not really forgot-
ten them."

One could see that M. was very close to tears during much of this
sharing. He then pulled himself together with the thought of how
brave they were. And then, from a deep, painful place in him, came
his "confession":

"I haven't got the guts they do — I couldn't live through that, not for
a day and certainly not years! I don't know how they made it — it
has to be a miracle. Maybe there is a God, but I haven't found
Him yet. My parents and their God found each other a long time
ago. I never wanted to hurt them when I realized I didn't believe,
when my faith began to come apart. Maybe it helped to be able to
talk to my father — he was certainly not old-fashioned. We could
talk about things he wanted for me, that he didn't have — an education, a chance to study in Israel, a chance to be on my own. I have
always loved adventure and always wanted more independence.
When I got to Israel and I started asking questions and the rabbis
didn't even know how to handle them, I started to become turned
off. First I made them uncomfortable, and then I made them ac-

tually nervous. I didn't get any answers, that's for sure! I was grappling with many issues and they weren't willing to grapple with me to help me, to be with me, or even to just let me be. I had to keep my mouth shut, and after awhile I felt ostracized. I just couldn't believe that a good and merciful God could allow so much evil to exist in the world. How could God let the Holocaust happen? I was so much more aware of the pain and suffering of the Holocaust in Israel—the people there have an incredible will to survive, to remember the past. I respect that, but my belief in traditional Judaism began to come apart, and I couldn't get it back together, and after awhile I stopped trying. I tried to hide it from my parents for a long time after I got back and I did a pretty good job, but it began to wear thin after awhile. During my whole college career I pretended I was orthodox. College certainly didn't help me revive my faith in traditional religion. What I saw in college helped put the finishing touches on any doubts I had about civilization. Not only the civilization that had produced the Holocaust, but one which was pushing the world toward a nuclear holocaust, a crazy society that had no respect for human values—the society seemed to be running amok. Why should I want to be a part of that? I tried so hard to learn to believe in myself—I yearned for *something* to believe in!"

I told M. that it seemed to me that he had searched for answers with integrity, and sometimes merciless and hopelessly painful integrity. I sensed that he was deeply sincere and sensitive *and* spiritual, and took life very seriously, when not running away from it. He was so overwhelmed by the pain of what he saw in the world and his parents' past. This pain was greatly exacerbated by his developmental problems, particularly his attempts at independence and his being the child of Holocaust survivors who had suffered many grievous losses and traumata.

I spent several sessions working on helping him discuss his pain and exploring both its personal, familial, and existential dimensions, and helping him acknowledge his pain as something respectable, related to very positive elements in himself as well as related to areas of difficulty. In addition, I confronted him with his own essential spirituality which was intense, even if overwhelmed with despair. At one point, I commented, "Don't you see how spiritual a person you really are? Nobody has a right to take that searching, spiritual quest from you, just as the Nazis didn't have the right to take it from your parents, and couldn't. No one will ever be able to take that from you!" M. felt very relieved after that, as if somehow he had once again joined the many generations of courageous Jews with whom he identified his parents, and their parents before them, and with whom he very much wanted to identify, and really didn't know he could.

With further confrontation and clarification as to the authenticity and value of his search and questions, in addition to many of the other factors of his personality which affected this, the therapy turned around very significantly. The ongoing sessions were extremely productive in terms of his ability to talk about details of his personal life including many things that previously would have proved embarassing. One of these things was the fact that he was taking money from his parents to subsidize his "non-income." We talked about his ambivalence to not working full-time or continuing with career development. He was able to share with me some of the dark experiences which had both philosophical and personal aspects, not only in terms of the horrors of the Holocaust and the death of so many million innocents, but his own feeling that *his* life was beyond hope and that *he* would end up a failure. After a number of sessions with strong confessional overtones, he was able to rally and get in touch with some positive life skills, his own natural enthusiasm, his hope for the future, his desire to make something of himself, and his trust in his own spirit. He learned that he did not *deny* God, but that he *challenged* God's reasons for letting all the evils occur.

At about this time the patient made a decision to go to California for a few months. This decision had escapist elements but also some strong elements of re-affirmation of life. He was once again in touch with a feeling for life, a desire for adventure, a passionate desire to engage with nature again, and to rediscover a sense of life's worthwhileness and purpose. He came back much energized. He had achieved many of the things we talked about as goals, and he began to see himself as reconnected to life. He decided to look again at his commitment to medicine by taking a volunteer job at a hospital. His difficulties about becoming involved in "our society" were circumvented by the fact that this was a volunteer program. He worked on an oncology program where he saw a great amount of terminal illness and a fair amount of death, and while he became discouraged some of the time, it was really a brave thing for him to do. One might call it "counterphobia with courage." He felt terrific about this. He moved forward toward rediscovering his early interest in medicine, this time in a much more authentic sense, in a clinical situation, facing the most tragic side of medicine. His ability to do this was a major accomplishment and re-confirmed the importance of giving him a sense of meaning and value in life.

As he moved forward in these areas, the relationship with his family gradually improved. We were able to hold some family sessions in spite of the parents' earlier reluctance. It was possible to help the parents and M. recognize how kindred they were in so many of their basic values. The following year M. went even further in his revived career interest by taking a graduate pre-med program and doing quite well, although some of his fears in a competitive situation diminished the overall lustre of his performance. M.'s earlier proclivity toward severe and debilitating, depressive episodes were greatly reduced and became much more manageable.

At the time of this writing we are still working on overcoming some of his fears of success, some of the traumatic second-generation effects of his parents' Holocaust experience, and some as yet unresolved self doubts and feelings of inadequacy. Mr. M. is now able to clearly affirm the value of being alive, for him and for the human race. While he still dislikes many features of general society, he no longer despairs. He sees himself as a spiritual person. He comfortably identifies himself as a Jew, somewhat heterodox in some of his beliefs, but accepts himself as nowhere as deviant as he thought he was. While his belief in a beneficent personal God has not re-emerged in the traditional sense, or in the form of adherence to the totality of orthodox Jewish practices, he has rediscovered for himself a more clear sense about God that has great positive value.

SUMMARY

The concept of a spiritual dimension can be a very useful and challenging concept in psychotherapy. It encompasses the psychic drive for integration, wholeness, balance, creative purpose in life, joy, episodes or a general state of expanded consciousness, a deep ethical sense and genuine conscience, and a capacity for unity and integration between one's self and the many relationships and commitments in one's life. The therapist's sense that there is a connection and unity among all these seemingly diverse elements often provides an additional useful framework for planning and conducting treatment. When the patient's sense of this dimension within himself emerges not as an artificial belief nor as an intellectual construct, but an inner experience of one's self, that inner experience often grows in extremely health-producing ways and seems to provide a source of energy.

For some patients, often but not always conventionally religious, the idea of God or a belief in or an experience of God seems similarly to be health-producing, especially if the therapist can work with it effectively. This relationship to God is often co-extensive with the elements of the "spiritual dimension."

The case provided here suggests some of the methods I have found useful in trying to apply this approach. I hope this case portrays the sense of energy and movement that can occur when the therapist helps the patient discover his own spiritual dimension. This sense of discovery is similar to insight but seems more encompassing and ultimately more far-reaching than traditional types of insights often tend to be.

The therapist facilitates this process by his openness to this domain of the psyche. It is wise to avoid the reductionism adherent in some current systems of psychotherapy. I suggest that the therapist does not summarily dismiss religious, philosophical, existential, and other potentially spiritual issues. Once the therapist begins to recognize the validity and usefulness of the spiritual dimension in the unfolding of the patient's personality, it begins to stand out more and more clearly even if grossly disguised and distorted by pathlogical forces. Psychotherapists of many schools recognize how extremely useful and vitally necessary is the therapist's own self-understanding. The same principle applies to the therapist's own spirituality and growth.

Chapter 8

A THERAPY OF RELIGIOUS IMAGERY FOR PARANOID SCHIZOPHRENIC PSYCHOSIS

DAVID T. BRADFORD, M.Th., Ph.D.

THE single case study is fertile ground theoretically. The sequence of feelings, ideas, images, and encounters may be traced, interrupted when appropriate with speculation and generalizations, and allowed continued flow within boundaries more natural than those drawn by controlled studies with large groups of subjects. The case study format also provides ready opportunity for presentation of individual characteristics of the patient and the special qualification of the psychotherapist who would work with more difficult cases. The present chapter focuses upon the psychotherapy of a young man bearing a diagnosis of paranoid schizophrenia who was preoccupied with religious "truths" derived from delusional beliefs, hallucinated almost continually about the haunting presence of religious figures, and implicitly cried out for companionship in his compact little world of religious madness.

An appropriate label for the therapeutic approach exemplified in this report would be "existential-phenomenological." The hyphen helps distinguish two richly diversified trends of European thinking about psychopathology and therapy which cohered first in the work of Ludwig Binswanger (1941-1942, 1957, 1960; May, Angel & Ellenberger, 1958; Needleman, 1963) and were later given expression in the research and psychotherapy of Van den Berg (1952-1953, 1972, 1975, 1980), Laing (1967, 1969), and others (Bradford, in

154

press; Spiegelberg, 1972). The specifically phenomenological trend is rooted in the work of Jaspers (1913/1963), Straus (1948, 1963, 1966, 1969), and Minkowski (1926, 1933/1970; Laing, 1963). The existential trend, which has always suffered a degree of obscurity due to the precariously bridged distance between the abstractions of existential philosphy and the pragmatics of clinical work, was somewhat slower in appearing, surfacing first in Binswanger's and later in Boss' work (1963; Scott, 1973,1975,1977).

In clinical work, allegiance to existential-phenomenological psychology requires passionate commitment to the basic humanity of even the most obnoxious and crazed patient; trust in the patient's ability to contribute in some measure to interpersonal encounter; and coolly reasoned examination and classification of even the most bizarre clinical phenomenology without thereby reducing these phenomena to pale outlines of a supposedly more "real" set of psychological factors. In sum, the existential-phenomenological approach may be described as humanistic, antireductionistic, and in a certain sense more a religious perspective that a psychological orientation.

When novel points of theory are presented in isolation from their germinal condition during actual therapeutic work, they often have a dryness which fails to do justice to the intensity of therapeutic involvement and the spontaneity with which these points and their associated interventions first came to light. For this reason, the present essay avoids an initial précis of relevant theory. Points of theory appear during the case presentation and thus are better understood as an integral feature of personal involvement with the patient. Following a brief history of the patient and the presentation of the four stages of psychotherapy, and a brief reflection on the clinical relevance of religious experience in schizophrenia, a synopsis of the principal interventions is offered in a final summary section.

THE PATIENT

The patient was a well built, blond-haired, 24 year-old Caucasian whose broad smile seemed the mark of a readiness for pleasure and fun despite the infrequency with which it interrupted his more typical glassy-eyed, dour expression. He was the oldest of three children and, aside from an "eccentric" aunt, the only family member with a psychiatric disturbance. Both parents were professional persons. He was quite popular in high school and was voted the vice-president of his senior class. His grades were sufficient for him to be admitted to a fine Ivy League university. He used marijuana and hallucinogens during his junior and senior year of high school and continued to do so during his freshman year of college. Midway through his first year of college, he came to believe the CIA was intent on enlisting him. Should he refuse to join their ranks, he believed, "they" would arrange for his grades to fall as well as for other forms of persecution. Frightened by these threats, he quit school, returned home, and enrolled in another university where once again the CIA intervened, further disrupting his life.

The patient experienced numerous conflicts with the legal authorities over the past 4 years. He had been jailed for indecency, vagrancy, and for causing a stir during suicide atempts he initiated in public. These periods of incarceration generally occurred following his escapes from mental hospitals or when he had impulsively decided to travel from home during periods of relative emotional stability. A final adventure, cut short by his most recent hospitalization at a state institution, was to have taken him to San Francisco's Golden Gate Bridge, from which his leap would create a final, dramatic splash.

The 4-year psychiatric history was extensive. With the exception of psychosurgery, the entire panoply of psychiatric treatments had been tried: milieu, art, and behavioral therapy, individual and group psychotherapy, psychotropic medicines, and a trial each of insulin and electroconvulsive therapy. A hospital progress note from the week prior to initiating psychotherapy spoke of the patient as "severly psychotic," "chronic," and having a "nuclear," unremitting kind of schizophrenia. The patient was unaware that because of his dangerousness hospital staff were talking of a permanent commitment to a maximum security facility.

During the 7 months (110 sessions) of our therapy, the patient's behavior changed to a degree which allowed him to accumulate a number of privileges. Initially he was allowed away from the locked ward only with staff supervision. Eventually he was allowed to roam the hospital grounds at will, noting his return on a roster at the nurses' station. Finally, he proved himself capable of holding a job in the hospital printing shop and was allowed to leave the hospital and visit downtown whenever he chose. Within a few weeks of the termination of therapy he interviewed for a halfway house placement in preparation for independent living, but failed to satisfy the interviewers' anxiety over his possible irresponsibility.

My involvement with the patient was arranged in a manner which made it unnecessary for me to participate in case conferences, confer privileges, or to speak with staff about the patient's behavior or medication. This is one of the few elements of experimental control which are available in single case studies in psychotherapy.

The pattern of progressively higher privileges stands roughly in an inverse relationship to the dosages and sedating properties of the medicines felt necessary for the patient during the 7 months of therapy. Two months prior to therapy he had been prescribed Mellaril, 100 *mg* daily, and lithium carbonate, 600 *mg* in the morning and 900 before sleep. During the first month of therapy the lithium was retained and the Mellaril raised to 300 *mg* b.i.d. Two months into therapy the lithium was discontinued. And 2 months later he began self-medication with Mellaril, 300 *mg* before sleep.

THE FIRST STAGE

To begin forming a relationship with a mad patient is to feel oneself sitting within a vacuum just ready to implode. There was little conversation, at best mere fragments of sentences spinning across a small room gradually filling with smoke from the patient's tobacco. A disorder of thinking partitioned the content of each of his phrases from that of its neighbors, thus warping and, finally, destroying the even flow and coherence of ordinary conversation.

Beneath the fragmented surface of the patient's conversation during the first stage of therapy were tides of emotion, currents of sundry feelings, and an inner array of sights and sounds for which the patient was a privileged audience. He was easily distracted and

had such poor concentration as a consequence of the welter of
private experience that he could have been described as a functional
mute blind to the world of ordinary reality and deaf to its words of
common sense. Yet there remained traces of his involvement with
another, psychotic world: the skin flushed occasionally, the pupils di-
lated, the corners of the mouth tuned upward, the body shifted. The
latter were reflections of psychosis; they manifested the body's dis-
quiet, its swelling, shifting, and changing postures under pressure
from forces foreign to the common world of sanity. The desired goal
of the first stage of therapy is that the therapist learn, rehearse in-
ternally, and come to know the characters and dramas of the patient's inner life. The therapist passively enters the patient's world,
as would an anthropologist intent upon recording the strange rituals
of a primitive tribe, or a cartographer plotting the eery landscape of
an alien planet.

The initial barrier to forming a therapeutic relationship was the
fragility of the patient's attention. Had he not been made aware of
how severely it truncated our conversation — or if he had become
testy and obtuse over having this called to his attention, instead of
feeling remorse over the poor quality of his concentration — therapy
could not have proceeded, much less have proved successful. Thus,
my early focus was with small but necessary details such as the quality of the patient's attention and the need for sustained concentration. This was done with such remarks as, "Something seems to be
stealing your attention. May I point out such moments when they
occur?" Eventually this will become, "Who are you talking with today?" or "Do your voices become upset when we discuss this?" The
flow of conversation commenced with the patient's commitment to
heightened attention, yet little was heard of the ordinary world for
two months, it having been substituted with the rich complexity of
the private world of psychosis.

Of paramount importance for the first stage of therapy was the
discovery of the patient's misuse of certain words meant to identify
the forms of perception associated with his psychotic experience. In
recounting his hallucinations and delusions, his intrusive thoughts
and nocturnal dreams, he would say, "I heard" when in fact he had
been thinking, "I dreamed" when he had envisioned, and "I had a vi-

sion" when he had actually been dreaming. Descriptions of voices, visions, and delusions were given with absolute assurance, but riddled with confusion over their respective perceptual modalities. The patient required training in recognizing and distinguishing the sources for the kinds of information which provided the intellectual and perceptual substance of his world. To this end, I introduced to the patient the idea of there being different sources of information, each associated with a different kind of knowledge.

For my patient, there were five sources of information: "voices" or auditory hallucinations; "visions" or visual hallucinations; "thoughts," which appeared spontaneously and raced autonomously through occasional vacancies of consciousness; "dreams" occurring during sleep; and perceptions involving any of the five ordinary senses and having for content the objects of the ordinary world. The first four provided substance for the patient's private world; the fifth was easily confused with the others. But with repeated questioning and frequent clarification on the part of the therapist, he came to know the distinctive, phenomenological marks of each.

The practical importance of the patient's bringing order to this perceptual confusion was not realized fully by him until later. When considering his possible placements outside the hospital during the third stage of therapy, he remarked that he would live in a commune established recently by former high school friends. I questioned his source for knowing of such a commune, meeting a condescending smile over asking such a silly question. If he misperceived the basis for this knowledge, I said, supposing it were relevant for the ordinary world when in fact it wasn't, there would be serious problems. He recanted, identified his source as a voice, and said, "It's true, there isn't such a place."

To question the source of one's information is to ask about the forms of thinking and perception, not the content conveyed through these means. Questions of truth and falsity, as they pertain to the content of the patient's delusions and hallucinations, are strictly prohibited from influencing the therapist's contribution to the relationship during the first stage. His role is simply to educate the patient by serving as a living primer in the epistemology of psychotic experience.

The structure of my patient's world may be described as a hierarchy composed of various levels of imagery and split from top to bottom by a deep rift paralleling his self-imposed segregation from the world of sanity and his own self-alienation. The multiple levels of imagery encompassed religious, political, artistic, and other figures. The dramas played with religious figures and their respective mythological props were the simplest and most easily understood, though the same designs were worked on lower levels by analogous figures. To the one side of the hierarchy was Christ Himself in the form of the patient; along with Christ were Harry Truman and Lyndon Johnson, Albert Schweitzer and Albert Einstein, André Malraux and Ken Kesey, and the Symbionese Liberation Army, a revolutionary band of urban guerillas which "fights totalitarian regimes," the patient said, and which dates from the onset of his psychosis. At the other end of the hierarchy were Satan—the patient's personal enemy—and Hitler and Mussolini, John F. Kennedy and Che Guevera, and Charles Manson and the punk rock star Johnny Rotten.

Figures from the two sides engaged in skirmishes and promoted each other's covert intrigues. Neither side yielded, nor had there been a "showdown" which demanded the patient's entire allegiance or compromised his inflated vanity. This would come later, though already during the first stage of therapy traces of resolution of the conflicts intrinsic to the structure of the hierarchy became apparent. For example, my patient announced apropos of nothing during an early conversation: "I saw the archangel Gabriel charge into Hell with the blessing of Heaven"; and then a few moments later: "Montezuma is meeting Cortes or one of his officials."

The first stage of therapy culminated with an experience which may be entitled "the shared psychotic tableau." It served to wed patient and therapist, binding them with a ring which circumscribed the patient's world, containing it, as never before, within the confines of a personal relationship. With my patient, the experience of the shared psychotic tableau was anticipated by several other, minor experiences which demonstrated my awareness of his special perspective. An example would be our conversation about his self-mutilation just prior to the most recent hospitalization. He had attempted to circumcise himself with a butcher knife while alone at home. The blood frightened his grandmother when she came to visit, and he threatened her when she called the police. I remarked in passing that he must have wanted to purify himself, to which he responded with shock, "Yes! How did you know?" With an accumulation of such experiences, the patient became more trusting; he relaxed in his madness, talked more freely, and unwittingly moved toward the moment of sharing.

Toward the end of one session the patient urged me excitedly to come outdoors. Ordinarily I am cautious to avoid interruptions, preferring to conduct therapy according to a plainly stated timetable and in a preestablished location with a specified seating arrangement. But the novelty of the patient's enthusiasm—the child-like wish to share with one's friend, if not one's father, a wonderful sight—was an unavoidable invitation. I stood, he led me outdoors, and with joyful humility which graded into tearful piety, he pointed to the three barren oak trees aligned on closely cropped brown grass against a dreary winter sky. These were the trees on which Jesus, Judas, and John the Baptist had been crucified. He knew this, having witnessed their communal crucifixion. The vision had been kept secure, harbored, accruing vividness in the privacy of the patient's madness, and now, for the first time, had been shared. He spoke coherently with lengthy sentences; he tripped over his words; he was warmed, and warmed me, with a vision eliciting a sense of holiness. This was the site of the world's redemption, the site where justice was brought to bear on the ancient crime betraying the best, the site where a righteous ascetic was punished for condemning the immorality of worldliness. Here, the patient's loneliness was broken, his isolation surmounted, his charity acknowledged by my willingness to receive his gift of a powerful, religious vision. The therapist who participates in such an experience will indeed have received a gift, but not without skirting hesitantly the cool rim of madness.

THE SECOND STAGE

If the first stage of therapy can be described as the therapist passively entering the psychosis, the second can be characterized by his actively engaging the figures of the pateint's private world and encouraging him to do the same. Passivity in the face of psychosis characterizes most psychotically disturbed schizophrenic patients. They may envision dragons and bear the assaults of Satan, but they seem never to take up St. George's lance or to make sure that Lucifer plummets, as Luke says, like the morning star. Such patients are often cowards, their occasional violence counterbalanced by timidity in the face of their own demons. A goal of the second stage is to counteract this cowardice. The patient must be taught to take his psychosis seriously. Knowing the patient's private world, the therapist is well prepared for this educational endeavor. Having the patient's trust, the therapist is able to offer encouraging goads as the patient is sent to battle.

For the patient to take action, his private world must be conceived as just that — a world: an integrally structured microcosm populated with its own *dramatis personae*, pervaded with its own set of moods and their respective geographies, and ordered in accordance with rules predicated by the "science" of magical, schizophrenic thought. To press home this idea of the patient living an independent and tightly structured, if not claustrophobic, world, I introduced the idea of there being two worlds — an extraordinary, spiritual world and an ordinary world of consensual validation, each of them coherent to a degree which allows only minimal interaction. This was done without fanfare or technicality, as if the idea was an afterthought one naturally would expect the patient to accept wholeheartedly. And he did so without reservation, thus reflecting with tacit approval that his existence was structured dualistically, divided sharply between the ordinary, phenomenal world of common sense and another, esoteric world visited by angels and demons, historical figures living and dead, and mapped repeatedly by the voices and epiphanies of God and His incarnate Son.

This perspective was eminently practical for the second stage of therapy since it promoted a sharp distinction between the patient's world, which heretofore he had confused horribly with the ordinary world, and the commmon sense world which grounds the experience of most persons. This perspective also allowed the patient to retain his world free from threats of skepticism projected by a "realistic" therapist inured to the mind-boggling impact of schizophrenic experience. The groundwork was thus layed for the patient and therapist to join one another in the other world, two allies defended by the therapist's discernment. An instance of this alliance during the second stage occurred when the patient noted with almost clairvoyant schizophrenic sensitivity that I was particularly tense during a session. I confessed to having my life threatened by another patient earlier in the day. Upon hearing this, he scowled, shifted in his seat, and announced that he was going to the ward at that moment to defend me.

Much else followed from the idea of there being two worlds. Since the patient was coming to fuller awareness of there being different sources of information, he was now prepared to learn that some sources of information pertain unalterably to one world while other sources pertain to a different world. Should he confuse worlds, assuming an otherworldly source for information issuing from the ordinary world, he would court confusion. As a consequence, he was called to note carefully when he passed inadvertently from one world to another. Similarly, he was called to maintain increased vigilance for the trickery and deceit of spirits which seem to speak from the ordinary world when, in fact, they were merely denizens of the other world.

To have adopted the two-world perspective was to expose himself to a range of feelings avoided psychotically. Once the patient recognized the existence of two worlds and began to adapt himself to the ordinary, he felt the sadness and nostalgia of losing his roots in the frightfully rich complexity of psychosis while simultaneously he experienced the arc of hope which transcended his narcissism and tied him to the unfulfilled promise that his investment in the ordinary world would compensate for this loss. By the same token, his recognizing the existence of two worlds and finding the ordinary one with its demands and narrow forms of consciousness intruding more and more on the even continuity of his psychotic experience, led him to recoil angrily from the encroachments of the ordinary world. Tension of this nature was often great; the patient resorted to the most grandiose ideas and became prone to the most outlandish behavior, "backsliding" like the early Roman Christians who chose martyrdom when the power, beauty, and ethos of their heavenly home was challenged.

An experience resting on acceptance of the two-world idea and embodying the call for action set forth in the second stage occurred

midway through a session when the patient's conversation was interrupted suddenly by a particularly severe distraction. I questioned
him; he responded that Satan had just entered the room and was
preparing to assume a definite shape. A lackadaisical expression
conveyed his skepticism toward my sincerity in suggesting we battle
Satan, but without my having time to respond, the patient tensed,
straightened in his chair, and appeared frightened. Since Satan's
form was shifting and growing, nearly filling our little office, I
pressed the patient to give a detailed description. Immediately following his description, Satan assumed the definite form of a large
"S"-shaped snake with green scales and a wry, sarcastic smile. The
patient pushed back against his seat and reported the snake's message with a mystified, startled expression. The words were identical
to the refrain of a popular song which puts this question in the
Devil's mouth: "Who do you think you're fooling?" I told the patient
to command Satan to remain stationary while he drew a picture of
the snake. With this done, I told him to command Satan to enter the
picture. I suggested a spear be used for the kill and had the patient
draw himself stabbing the beast, which he did, further mocking Satan by drawing a handlebar mustache on the snake. Finally, I tore
the snake's foot from the drawing and suggested the patient destroy
it. I took the remainder, saying that I, too, would destroy my part.
He smiled, then laughed victoriously, suggesting that perhaps the
toilet would be an appropriate repository.

Satan embodied the great doubt; he was the persistently poised,
delicately manipulated pin which threatened to burst the patient's
bubble of psychosis. Satan was the thorn in the patient's side. Satan
knew a secret which the patient kept private. Satan questioned the
patient's self-assured commitment to the other world. Satan was an
acrid gas capable of rendering unpalatable and poisonous the thin
air of the patient's Icarian flight. Satan knew someone was fooling
himself. Satan was poised to spring; the therapist would only have to

shift his interpretation of the other world, such that it became the patient's own world rather than an extraordinary world of purely transcendental proportions, for Satan to spring forward, filling the therapist.

What purpose was served by battling Satan? Would it not have proved more helpful to cultivate Satan's presence and to entertain seriously his question to the patient? Such a frontal attack on the patient's self-deception would have proved disastrous for the therapeutic relationship. The therapist would instantly have become the Evil One himself, his disclaimers viewed by the patient as no more convincing than Judas' claim to innocence. No, a frontal attack is not allowed, even skirmishes are to be avoided prior to the third stage of psychotherapy. Instead, the therapist and patient must work together to tighten the psychosis, to render easily discernible the differences between the kinds and sources of information pertaining to the two worlds, and generally to enhance the patient's ability to adapt at will to either one. Without success in these endeavors, improvements in the patient's condition would have represented groundless accommodations to behavioral demands he felt were superficial. This world of ordinary reality, however dull or threatening, must be viewed by the patient as safe; and for it to be so viewed, he must know the therapist as an ally who moves with facility in either world, teaching and modeling a manner of doing so. A satanic therapist would have created enmity in the patient, thus tipping the scale in favor of his fear of the ordinary world and his retreat to psychosis from the fresh demands accompanying his adaptation to this world. The intention of the present style of therapy is not to repress or destroy the psychosis, but rather to reduce severely its valence in the interplay of psychosis and normality.

THE THIRD STAGE

I introduced the third stage of therapy by commenting, as if with an aside of relative unimportance, that the spiritual world was the patient's personal world. The "other" world would now be "his" world. Demons could haunt, God speak, and the dead live, but they would do so in a psychic world of the patient's own. Interpretations were made in these terms, and they roused ire which remained mostly unabated for weeks. Now I was the dull ignoramus who "wouldn't recognize Christ if he walked up to you on the street unless he was wearing a toga!" Were I not so self-satisfied and un-enlightened, I would see Christ was sitting across the table from me. I was like the rest — like his father, like the doctor, like the staff, like an adult, all of them mindlessly entrenched in their mundane world.

Anger marked the patient's entrance into the third stage of psychotherapy. I recall my fear when he returned from a moment of distraction and announced suddenly and with a wide-eyed, maniacal anger approximating the righteous indignation of the psalmist's god that he was Jesus Christ. There was danger for the therapist now since the patient's anger toward him was proportionate to his love. And yet this was also the stage during which reminiscences of the patient's personal history first emerged, vastly enlarging the scope of interpretive interventions.

Upon entering the third stage of psychotherapy, the therapist is called to supplement with material from the patient's personal history the imaginal hierarchy constructed during the first stage, noting analogies between the activities of psychotic figures and the dramas once enacted by parents, friends, and family. He is also called to move up and down the entire hierarchy, drawing upon multiple levels of imagery in order for an interpretation to promote a convincing insight with emotional weight. The movement of conversation may be halting and tentative during the third stage, occasionally veering into delusional material, but the patient's attention is obtained and kept more easily, and he is better able to tolerate emotional intensity without the unusually severe distractions.

Three examples of experience from this stage will provide a sense of the patient's concerns, the way different levels of imagery interpenetrate, and the style of therapeutic intervention. Each involves father-like figures of different, and sometimes opposing, characteristics.

The patient sat bolt upright in his chair with a startled expression and announced that 30 minutes prior to that very moment Hitler had been killed in a local Lion's Club. The source of information was "thought"; the image, political. When asked how he felt, the patient said, "Elated!" And with good reason: Hitler was dead, the Third Reich ended. Hitler had been a most elusive criminal, escaping from his bunker, from Nuremberg, from Alcatraz. He had been disguised as the socialist, John F. Kennedy, and he was the very beast of the New Testament's Book of the Revelation. With his death, a critical victory was scored over the disruptive forces of the evil side of the hierarchy. More important for practical purposes, and with bearing on the worldly activities of the patient, was the death of one whose government represented an unsuccessful, repressive, and socialistic answer to the disheartening bankruptcy of a crushed republic. Was it an accident, I asked rhetorically, that Hitler was killed on the day the patient was anxious and disheartened over the possibility of losing his job due to a work-related oversight? As Hitler proved the enemy of fiscal stability and national morale, his death provided the encouragement and assurance needed for the patient to apologize for his oversight and request of his supervisor a fresh assignment at work.

The second example involved the patient's feeling that he was the father of everyone on the ward, then several days later envisioning himself raising Elvis Presley from the grave. Elsewhere (Bradford, 1980) I have discussed the lore surrounding Elvis' death and shown its similarity to the mythological presentation in the Gospels of Jesus Christ's death, resurrection, postmortem appearances, and ascension. From this perspective, the patient's feeling of fathering the ward and his vision of raising Elvis provide a window onto a deep-seated psychotic process which promoted the patient's identification with a creative father-god to the end that the patient himself, in the guise of a popular savior who rode a crest of drugs and popularity into the tomb, might be raised, intact and psychologically resuscitated.

The final example was decidedly more personal that the preceding two. With disavowal of personal responsibility and with a tone which conveyed shame, the patient reported a dream which had occurred on the eve of his last visit home. The dream was meaningless, he said, and not his own creation. In the dream, he impulsively rushed toward a large, white bust of my head and planted dynamite at its base. From beside the statue, I commented musingly, "This must be countered," but only stroked my chin and seemed to invite him to destroy it. The dynamite exploded. The patient felt terribly confused and rushed about trying to patch together the pieces.

The dream analysis began with my asking simply, "Are you apologizing for having hard feelings toward me?" He replied, "That's exactly what I'm doing!" and proceeded to talk spontaneously of my difference from his own father, who had not tolerated such hard feelings. I assured him of my understanding how he might both like and dislike me. Shortly thereafter his shame over the dream received attention. He felt ashamed of being a mental patient, and, once released, he would note carefully whether to share this information with a given person. Similarly, he felt humiliated and disgusted with himself upon visits home. He visited, not because he missed either his home or his parents—he hated both—but because this was his only means of leaving the hospital. As a consequence of pursuing such visits, he felt his self-reliance and personal integrity were compromised. But the discovery and expression of these intimate feelings were not so surprising or thrilling to him as was another, quite different kind of experience toward the end of the conversation. He rose from his normal, stooped position, looked at me eye-to-eye with a shocked expression, and said, "I heard my voice." It became clear after a few questions that the patient had heard his own speaking voice for the first time in years.

THE FOURTH STAGE

The final stage of therapy developed as the patient became more able to converse on topics pertaining to both the ordinary and his own world without showing an especially strong preference for material specific to his unique perspective. Additional marks of the patient's readiness to enter the fourth stage were his willingness after having been distracted by intrusive thoughts to be redirected to conversation focusing on ordinary matters, and his capacity to extend and develop conversation by drawing upon ordinary associations rather than psychotically derived ideas. By this time, he met the tensions of therapy mostly with ordinary coping skills. He might cringe with anger, smirk with sarcasm, mention his affections and dislikes, and actively resist as would a stubborn child, all without slipping into the glazed, passive expression of dulled conformity with his circumscribed madness. With his heightened attention and better concentration, sessions had become lengthier, some lasting for 50 minutes.

I initiated formally the fourth stage of psychotherapy largely by ignoring psychotic material and giving special attention to the interpersonal and vocational chores of daily life. This would have been simply a behavioral program utilizing extinction technique were it not for the exceptional moments when a particularly severe distraction of the patient's attention signalled the need for careful delineation of the source and meaning of an intrusive thought or voice. Psychotherapy was now a two-pronged endeavor. On the one hand, there was counseling about matters pertaining to interpersonal and vocational success in the ordinary world; on the other, there was the effort, immediately following the increasingly rare moments of distraction, to broaden the scope of interpretive interventions by giving added attention to the psychodynamic features of the therapeutic relationship. To the information about his personal history provided by the patient during the third stage, I now added my slowly garnered conclusions about dynamically structured patterns of the therapeutic relationship and similarly structured dramas enacted by figures from various levels of the psychotic hierarchy. Often interpretations failed to carry the emotional impact and the intuitive certainty which an interpretation conveys under best of circumstances. And yet the technique of multileveled interpretation is not to be neglected: it promotes a further step in vitiating the psychosis, without thereby dissolving its tight boundaries, by enabling the patient to recognize and to acknowledge on a rational basis the similarities between the psychotic drama and the personal dramas of his ordinary life.

An instance of multileveled interpretation occurred during the final stage of therapy which resulted in a stunning and remarkably comprehensive insight on the part of the patient. We were speaking about the question of whether a woman "owns" a man, or vice versa.

Shortly we came to personal material. Yes, his mother — or rather his stepmother, since the patient believed he was adopted by a witch disguised as the natural mother — owned his father, just as the patient himself had been owned or controlled by her. Conversation progressed smoothly from this point until the patient began having a difficult time concentrating. When I asked the cause of his distraction, he reported trying to carry on three conversations at once: one with Moses, one with a dead man trying to escape from a coffin, and a third with an old girl friend who for some weeks had been an important focus of his thinking. At that specific moment he had been arguing with the girl over which of them owned the other.

The quality of the patient's involvement with his world deepened suddenly. He reported a particularly lucid fantasy of a large figure resembling a corroded Greek statue with empty eye sockets. The statue was inhabited by the fleeting ghost of a dead woman, and at its base lay a man whose feeling was sad resignation over his state of affairs. The prostrate man found it an awful and unanticipated surprise to experience death as he then was.

My interpretation commenced with a simple remark. "Sounds autobiographical," I said, to which the patient responded, "Explain what you mean." I drew upon the fantasy at hand and supplemented it with material from discussions of the figures most recently active in the patient's world. "The hollow-eyed statue — that's how you look when you're distracted. As for the ghost — is she any different from the feminine voice we talked about the other day, that woman with so many sides who lies to you and humiliates you? She's the one who would own you, the one who tries to take hold of you like the ghost does the statue. And the man laying beneath the statue...I wonder if you haven't felt the same?" Gesturing around our tiny office to indicate the patient's entire experience of hospitalization, I said, "After all, how much of all this did you permit to happen?" With an uneven tone of surprising quietness for a person so self-assured and affirmative, the patient said, "I used to be able to do that kind of analysis with a book, but for some reason I haven't been able to do it with myself." I suggested he consider his private world as a book, to which he responded with conviction, "Yes! Literary analysis on my thoughts!"

Here, then, is an insight into his very lack of insight. For the patient to have glimpsed the flawed character of his self-understanding, he must have adopted, if only momentarily, a perspective sufficiently objective to question, criticize, and, eventually, to doubt the authority of his psychosis. The Christ-like madman had evidently rubbed shoulders with the satanic snake which once asked, "Who do you think you're fooling?"

DISCUSSION OF TECHNIQUE

The fourth stage of psychotherapy is interminable. Just as the self-possession of the spiritually mature cracks under the existential crises which bow all persons, even more does one expect relapses and crises in the personality of a young man whose development had been truncated by schizophrenic psychosis. By the same token, less is to be expected from the partially healed schizophrenic person who attempts adaptation to the working places of the ordinary world. My patient's 5-year allegiance to a world of demons and spirits had been as the lifelong, waking dream of a monk interned in some bizarre monastery. One does not awaken easily; and once awake, there is another order of existence requiring careful study and counsel. That wakefulness is possible in such cases is demonstrated by the outline of behavioral changes presented earlier in this essay.

Those who have relegated the riddle of schizophrenia to the neurochemical laboratory might expect the patient's improvement to be short-lived, his stability and relative clear-headedness faltering soon after the termination of psychotherapy. But this neglects the directional, if not teleological nature of some forms of schizophrenic psychosis. Perry (1974) and others (Bateson, 1974; Boisen, 1960; Epstein, 1979; Gunderson, 1980; Horton, 1973; Matthews, Roper, Mosher & Menn, 1979) have made abundantly clear the processional nature of such illnesses, showing their coherence and intrinsic power to adjust the psychological distortions of the conscious personality. Evidence for this was apparent from several conflicts which occupied my patient during the fourth stage of psychotherapy.

The first conflict involved his delusional identification with

Christ. This had been a matter-of-fact item of belief duirng the initial two stages of therapy; it was defended vociferously and began to weaken during the third; and was a subject for rational criticism during the fourth. How could he be Christ, the patient queried, when he no longer wanted to bear the sins of those dear to him, including myself. On the other hand, he reflected, should he forgive and trust, he would implicitly grant them license to sin again, thereby jeopardizing his righteous, deceptively tranquil role of divine omnipotence.

Another conflict involved his understanding of the reason for his hospitalization. During earlier stages of therapy, he believed his problems stemmed from being tricked into taking dozens of tablets of an hallucinogenic drug. The drug was somehow different and stronger than the one he requested. With the strange, mathematical wizardry which schizophrenic persons muster often, he had calculated the exact day in the future when the drug effect would disappear. Then, late in the fourth stage of therapy, he asked, "Why am I in the hospital? I've been told I'm 'Schizophrenia, Paranoid,' but that doesn't mean anything to me," to which I replied, "You're unable to get along socially on the outside, not well enough to take care of yourself." His response: "Get along socially, huh? That's the first explanation that's made any sense to me. Well, I can't be day dreaming out in public!"

The third conflict was engendered purely by the psychosis; its instigation did not require an intervention, nor did it rest on the patient adopting initially an idea at variance with the psychosis. He rose from his seat and announced that Krishna had just told him that "contacts" as well as mediumistic "communications" with the dead were undesirable, and that the former should be avoided altogether. "Contacts," he explained, were visions, while "communications" were a matter of listening to voices. He felt this was sound advice which he would follow, and I agreed, remarking upon the Indian stories which emphasize Krishna's mastery of ordinary life. Madness may be said to raise above its own tumult a banner proclaiming hope of liberation. Krishna's dictum was such a banner; its inscription, a therapeutic intervention on the part of madness itself.

RELIGIOUS EXPERIENCE AND SCHIZOPHRENIA

The madman's religious experience poses an impressive barrier to his therapist's understanding. The reasons are many, pertaining to the therapist's own kind of religiousness, the particular philosophical stance embodied in the discipline which shaped his training, and not least important, the patent oddity of schizophrenic symptomatology. The assertions, rebuttals, and rejoinders traded by Bergin (1980a, 190b), Ellis (1980), and Wells (1980) reflect the significance of the therapist's own religiousness for psychotherapy. Scholarly humility dictates a somewhat naive approach to so complex an area, and common sense would have one suspect that the crazed patient knows his religious experience, and even its bearing for therapy, as well as the therapist, whose anchor of sanity preserves him from the tidal force of religious madness.

The boundaries marking the area of investigation must be drawn tightly, otherwise the entire effort floats uneasily under the influence of ideas without experiential content. For purposes of clarity, only the patient's experience of God will be considered. Excluded are visions and voices and eery perceptual distortions created by demons, spirits, and saints, enthusiastic spoutings of prophecy, the commandeering of one's body by accomplices acting in concert with the dead, and any number of other, similarly nontheistic experiences. Excluded as well are dogmatic assertions pertaining to the properly theological content of the term "God," and also interpretations resting on psychology and psychiatry's own metaphysic of "archetype," "superego," or other structures and processes alleged to be responsible for religious madness. The research question addressed to the patient must be simple, and the method of reporting his reponse, and reflecting upon its bearing for therapy and for the therapist personally, must be equally simple and straightforward. The following paragraphs detail the response of three schizophrenic patients to the question, "Tell me of your experience of God, the first such experience which comes to mind." Interpretive comments are minimal, and philosophically critical remarks are dealt sparingly.

I believe these three patients are representative of the wide spectrum of theistic experiences in schizophrenically disturbed individuals. To one extreme is Anthony, surely one of the most charismatic persons I have met. To the other extreme is the patient of the preceding case study. About midway is Mary. Anthony's experience is relentlessly monotheistic, and could have been composed by Sharafuddin Maneri (Jackson, 1980) or another devotional mystic of Islam with an equally radical theology of transcendence. The patient of the present case study more closely resembles a pantheist, though certainly not of the expansive, charitable, humane variety capable, as was Wordsworth (1886), of discerning the "motion and spirit" which "dwells in the light of setting suns," "rolls through all things," and lightens the "burden... of all this unintelligible world." Mary is different from both in that her experience of God recalls the gracious deity of the Judao-Christian tradition whose transcendent presence becomes immanently focused in certain historical occurrences.

During adolescence, and rather infrequently thereafter, one meets individuals whose personal charisma and ethical integrity create an enduring effect. Such was the case with the frail-boned Anthony, a red-haired, blue-eyed, light-complected troubadour. He had been committed by an Episcopal priest because of the disturbance the patient's outdoor preaching caused the parishioners as they approached the parking lot after Sunday services. He actually sang beautifully, and recited psalms from memory as he waited for meals in the decidedly foul air of a state hospital ward filled with mentally disturbed ghetto residents. An aura of sweetness, as with incense, pervaded his presence. Others felt the same; rather than hound him, beg food or cigarettes from him, or ridicule his Anglo-Saxon pallor and religious fervor, he was mostly left alone. To describe his intensity clinically in terms of "affect" or "mood" would miss the point: his intensity was cool, one might say, in that it arose from a different source than the friction of interpersonal encounter; and yet hot, in the sense of posing a threat to those who would court false intimacy or attempt to elicit the quick repartee.

The experience reported by Anthony occurred on the psychiatric ward of the county hospital before he was transported to the state facility. He was standing in front of a barred window when he saw the setting sun split into many pieces, forming a beautiful pattern of bright, dancing fragments. Forms like rocket ships exploded from the fractured orb, making the scene all the more impressive. A voice announced that the vision was of God, but Anthony doubted, and said, "If you're God, show me." Sufficicent proof was not forthcoming. Anthony turned away.

Anthony's report seems not to involve an experience of God *per se*. God's presence in the vision or in the voice was denied. Neither met the tacit criteria set by Anthony's "testing of the spirits." But it is precisely by merit of such negative findings with respect to God's appearance, and His meaning, that one is able to ascertain a positive notion of His possible appearances and His bearing for psychotherapy. Of foremost importance is Anthony's refusal to identify God with the fantastic and no doubt enormously powerful vision of the solar explosion or with the verbal announcement of this being God Himself. Anthony's religious stance may be characterized as iconoclastic in a comprehensive sense: not only does he refuse to identify God with a fantastic and powerful set of psychotically derived phenomena, but by extension one supposes that he would do the same should some less extravagant and less powerful, worldly image of God be proclaimed. For Anthony, the experience reveals God as a factor distinct from psychotic imagery, and perhaps separable from any possible image, regardless of one's mental condition or state of consciousness.

For the psychotic schizophrenic person, to be tied to such a God is to be liberated from emotional adherence to the intrusive visions and voices of an acute episode; and with the greater play of emotion allowed by such liberation, one's capacity to think coherently is enhanced as well. Of no small importance for those whose psychosis is compounded with paranoia, such an emotional and intellectual liberation may guard against the complicating and tightening of the paranoid system, given the lessened need to filter both psychotic and normal imagery in terms of the need for self-justification or punishment.

How could such an experience be other than heartening for the psychotic patient, and how could such a God be other than a mainstay for one wrestling with scrambled thinking and tumultuous feelings? Psychotherapy with a patient like Anthony does well to cultivate experience of such a God so long as the acute episode continues. Either during or after the episode, such experiences should be recalled and held before the patient as examples of his finest clarity and purest piety. And should the therapist himself be a quester of God, accounts such as Anthony's deserve to be placed in a hagiography of schizophrenic saints.

The second example is drawn from the main case study presented in this chapter. The patient was asked about his experience of God during a rather heated discussion about whether the other world of visions and voices was his own personal world. He resisted the idea mightily. He demanded a definition of the ordinary world, the one he fought to resist and would have loved to enter. I offered my working definition, describing the ordinary world as commonsensical, the norm, a kind of collection of material objects the identity of which was agreed upon through consensual validation. This was not his world, the patient said. Rather, his world was God, and God was his world. The two were identical. When asked to describe such an experience, he spoke of God as being "all around," as if "each thing were a part of God." He continued: "Now, I'm not saying I don't go to the store for cigarettes. I do. And I'm not saying that when I want a 'Coke,' I don't go to the machine to buy it. All of that kind of thing is so. But my experience is different from others'. Even the attendants — they don't understand it. I have my own view. I have my own thoughts, my own little world."

The specifically religious content of much of this patient's psychosis becomes understandable in the light of his report. For this young man, during the course of much of his illness, paranoid schizophrenic psychosis was an even continuity of otherworldly existence punctuated repeatedly by hierophanies. The case history attests to this, with its many gods, demons, angels, and spirits.

The final account is Mary's. She was an obese Caucasian in her mid-30s whose life had been interrupted several years before with the first of many schizophrenic episodes. Having lost her husband and two children to religious madness, she lived a constant shuttle between board and care homes and the psychiatric ward of a county hospital. God had spoken with her for years, and she treasured His infrequent and occasionally somewhat coquettish visitations. When asked about her experience of God, she responded as follows:

> I had been praying when God showed His feeling for me...Oh,
> my God, it was so beautiful! They were just His feelings, not my
> own—they could only come from Him. His feelings for me were
> good and beautiful, perfect, clean, and good. Just like when you
> had a baby, like when you take your son and hold him on your lap
> and squeeze him and love him and kiss him and he does it back to
> you. Then he feels your love for him, knows you love him. When
> God did that to me, it was His feelings toward me. I can't
> describe them. I didn't know what to do. I said out loud to Him,
> "I give it all back!" I went on and a couple of days later an angel
> came. A man was suddenly standing there—it was an angel—and
> he said, "You gave it all back." Then he disappeared.

The healing force and pristine beauty of Mary's experience seem
utterly transparent. Interpretive notions relying upon a hermeneutic
of faulty parenting, father and mother surrogates, infantile regression, defensively structured projections of unconscious needs, or any
number of other mediating concepts pale beside its simple reciproc-
ity and luxuriously fulfilling affectivity.

SUMMARY

The therapeutic approach illustrated in the case presented in the
body of this text involves 10 principal interventions. Without adduc-
ing the broader theoretical structure upon which these interventions
rest, they may be summarized as follows:

The first stage. (1) The fragility of the patient's concentration is
of utmost concern initially. Without his agreeing to the therapist calling him to attention gently and repeatedly, therapy simply cannot
proceed. (2) Shortly after therapy is initiated, the therapist intro-
duces the idea of there being different sources of information which
require careful and consistent demarcation. (3) Upon assuming a
passive stance, the therapist enters the world of psychosis, thereby
availing himself of the information needed for the re-creation of the
patient's multileveled and deeply confused psychotic hierarchy. (4)
One awaits the experience which signals the intimate alliance of

therapist and patient, and serves notice for beginning the second state. Following the experience of the shared psychotic tableau, the second stage is initiated.

The second stage. (5) The second stage commences with the therapist introducing the two-world idea, helping to differentiate for the patient both the ordinary world of consensual validation as well as another, extraordinary world populated with God and gods, the dead and living, and a panoply of other figures and voices. Different sources of information are assigned to their respective worlds, and the patient is pressed to recognize the practical implications of confusing his worlds. (6) With the therapist initially taking the lead, the patient is encouraged to act in his other world in a brave and decisive manner.

The third stage. (7) With the therapist's reinterpretation of the two-world idea, such that the "other" world is now the patient's own psychic world, the third stage commences. On the one hand, anger and possible danger mark the patient's greeting of this reinterpretation, while on the other, the richness of intimate, personal historical reminiscences may now enter therapy. The latter allows the therapist to supplement his re-creation of the psychotic hierarchy with information pertaining to the patient's personal history.

The fourth stage. (8) The marks of readiness for the final, interminable stage of psychotherapy are: heightened attention, lengthier concentration, a willingness following distraction to be redirected to conversation based on ordinary associations, the absence of preference for conversation based on psychotic material, a capacity to extend and develop conversation involving ordinary matters, and a reliance on skills common to the conversation of those who are sane. Upon its initiation, the therapist mostly ignores the psychosis. (9) This program of extinction is punctuated, however, with multi-leveled, interpretive interventions which draw upon the psychodynamics of the psychotic hierarchy, the patient's personal history, and the emotional patterning of the therapeutic relationship.

The tenth and final point upon which this style of therapy rests is the recognition and increasingly frequent cultivation of the healing force intrinsic to some forms of schizophrenic psychosis.

Freud recommended an emotional abstinence on the part of the couchbound psychoanalyst. The present style of therapy recommends an asceticism of the spirit which urges and preserves intellectual objectivity while harboring, and drawing upon, the passion intrinsic to the experience of religious madness.

REFERENCES

Bateson, G. (Ed.) *Perceval's Narrative: A Patient's Account of his Psychosis, 1830-1832.* New York: William Morrow, 1974.

Bergin, A.E. Psychotherapy and religious values. *Journal of Consulting and Clinical Psychology,* 1980, *48,* 95-105. (a)

Bergin, A.E. Religious and humanistic values. *Journal of Consulting and Clinical Psychology,* 1980, *48,* 642-654. (b)

Binswanger, L. Existential analysis, psychiatry, schizophrenia. *Journal of Existential Psychiatry,* 1960, *1,* 157-165.

Binswanger, L. On the relationship between Husserl's phenomenology and psychological insight. *Philosophy and Phenomenological Research,* 1941-1942, *2,* 199-210.

Binswanger, L. *Schizophrenie.* Pfullingen:Neske, 1957.

Boisen, A.T. *Out of the Depths: An Autobiographical Study of Mental Disorder and Religious Experience.* New York: Harper & Brothers, 1960.

Boss, M. *Psychoanalysis and Daseins-analysis* (L.B. Lefebre, Trans.). New York: Basic Books, 1963.

Bradford, D.T. *The Experience of God: Portraits in the Phenomenological Psychopathology of Schizophrenia.* New York: Peter Lang, in press.

Bradford, D.T. *A Structural Analysis of the Figure of Elvis.* Unpublished manuscript, 1980.

Ellis, A. Psychotherapy and atheistic values. *Journal of Consulting and Clinical Psychology,* 1980, *48,* 635-639.

Epstein, S. Natural healing processes of the mind: Acute schizophrenic disorganization. *Schizophrenia Bulletin,* 1979, *5,* 313-321.

Gunderson, J.C. A reevaluation of milieu therapy for nonchronic schizophrenic patients. *Schizophrenia Bulletin,* 1980, *6,* 64-69.

Horton, P.C. The mystical experience as a suicide preventive. *American Journal of Psychiatry,* 1973, *130,* 294-296.

Jackson, P. (Ed.) *Sharafuddin Maneri: The Hundred Letters.* New York: The Paulist Press, 1980.

Jaspers, K. *General Psychopathology* (J. Hoenig & M.W. Hamilton, Trans.). Chicago: University of Chicago Press, 1963. (Originally published, 1913.)

Laing, R.D. Minowski and schizophrenia. *Review of Existential Psychology,* 1963, *9,* 195-207.

Laing, R.D. *The Politics of Experience.* New York: Phantom Books, 1967.

Laing, R.S. *The Divided Self.* New York: Pantheon, 1969.

Matthews, S.M., Roper, M.T., Mosher, L.R. & Menn, A.Z. A non-neuroleptic treatment for schizophrenia: Analysis of the two-year post-discharge rate of relapse. *Schizophrenia Bulletin*, 1979, *5*, 322-333.

May, R., Angel, E. & Ellenberger, H.F. (Eds.) *Existence: A New Dimension in Psychiatry and Psychology*. New York: Simon & Schuster, 1958.

Minkowski, E. Bergson's conceptions as applied to psychopathology (F.J. Farnell, Trans.). *The Journal of Nervous and Mental Disease*, 1926, *63*, 553-568.

Minkowski, E. *Lived Time: Phenomenological and Psychopathological Studies* (N. Metzel, Trans.). Evanston, Ill.: Northwestern University Press, 1970. (Originally published, 1933.)

Needleman, J. (Trans.) *Being-in-the-World: Selected Papers of Ludwig Binswanger*. New York: Basic Books, 1963.

Perry, J.W. *The Far Side of Madness*. Englewood Cliffs, N.J.: Prentice-Hall, 1974.

Scott, C.E. Daseinsanalysis: An interpretation. *Philosophy Today*, 1975, *19*, 182-197.

Scott, C.E. Heidegger, madness, and well-being. *Southwest Journal of Philosophy*, 1973, *4*, 157-177.

Scott, C.E. (Ed.) *On Dreaming: An Encounter with Medard Boss*. Chico, Calif.: Scholars Press, 1977.

Spiegelberg, H. *Phenomenology in Psychology and Psychiatry: An Historical Introduction*. Evanston, Ill.: Northwestern University Press, 1972.

Straus, E.W. *On Obsession: A Clinical and Methodological Study*. New York: Nervous & Mental Disease Monographs (No. 78), 1948.

Straus, E.W. *Phenomenological Psychology: The Selected Papers of Erwin W. Straus* (E. Eng, Trans.). New York: Basic Books, 1966.

Straus, E.W. *Primary World of the Senses: A Vindication* (J. Needleman, Trans.). Glencoe, Ill.: Free Press, 1963.

Straus, E.W., Natanson, M. & Ey, H. *Psychiatry and Philosophy*. New York: Springer-Verlag, 1969.

Van den Berg, J.H. *A Different Existence: Principles of Phenomenological Psychopathology*. Pittsburgh, Penn.: Duquesne University Press, 1972.

Van den Berg, J.H. The human body and the significance of human movement. *Philosophy and Phenomenological Research*, 1952-1953, *13*, 159-183.

Van den Berg, J.H. On hallucinating: Critical-historical overview and guidelines to further study. *Journal of Phenomenological Psychology*, 1975, *6*, 1-16.

Van den Berg, J.H. Phenomenology and psychotherapy. *Journal of Phenomenological Psychology*, 1980, *2*, 21-49.

Wells, G. Values and psychotherapy. *Journal of Consulting and Clinical Psychology*, 1980, *48*, 640-641.

Wordsworth, W. Lines, composed a few miles above Tintern Abbey, on revisiting the banks of the Wye during a tour. In M. Arnold (Ed.), *Poems of Wordsworth*. London: Macmillan, 1886.

Chapter 9

RELIGIOUS IMAGERY IN THE PSYCHOTHERAPY OF A BORDERLINE PATIENT

ROBERT J. LOVINGER, Ph. D.

INTRODUCTION

SOME therapists regard the presence of a significant religious orientation in the patient as an aberration or at least a nuisance (Ellis, 1970, 1978, 1980) or as irrelevant or private to both patient and therapist (Fromm-Reichmann, 1950, p. 33). On the other hand, some have expressed varying degrees of positive expectation toward the patient's religious orientation, such as Jung who took an existential view of religion and those who express a welcoming attitude to the emergence of religious sentiment in therapy (Evans, 1973; Vayhinger, 1973), and still others who view the expression of religious belief as a nearly crucial part of therapy (Adams, 1970). Other therapists work religious issues into treatment only when necessary. The collaboration between an ordained rabbi (also a clinical psychologist) with a psychiatrist (Kagan & Zucker, 1970) has been reported, but this is apparently not common. In varying ways, many psychotherapists have accepted that it is important to consider the religious patient's orientation and concerns in therapy (Atwood, 1974; Beit-Hallahmi, 1975; Coyle & Erdberg, 1969; Oates, 1950; Pruyser, 1971, 1977; Rizzuto, 1979; Spero; 1981).

Psychotherapists have been slow to develop adequate means to evaluate and treat religious patients who request treatment. Indeed, most therapists who received their training in secular institutions have no background in clinical work with or even theoretical approaches to religious issues in psychotherapy other than personal knowledge and experience. This is partly because the patient's religious background is rarely regarded as deserving special consideration — a curious attitude given the proportion (well over 80 percent) of the American population that regards itself as religious. Therapists are often puzzled as to what to do when religious issues surface in therapy or what theoretical models may be useful with such problems. Further, the highly personal, and often very positive or negative valences of psychotherapists toward religion (Ragan, Malony, & Beit-Hallahmi, 1980) may leave the therapist particularly vulnerable to the evocation of countertransference reactions stemming from personal, cultural, and professional sources (Lovinger, in press). While these problems will not be elaborated upon here, suffice it to say that the potential for countertransference reactions in the therapist, the paucity of systematic knowledge in the area of religion, and the fact that most of the American population practices some form of religion or maintains some specific religious beliefs, all combine to indicate that religion can have a profound impact on therapy even if the patient never mentions it. Patients are very astute — they won't mention religion if they think the therapist does not want to hear about it.

The therapist's personal background, training, theoretical orientation, and technique all impact on how religion is handled in therapy. The therapist's interaction with religious patients is also effected by demographic variables. Therapists working in a community mental center in a highly conservative, Southern or Southwestern milieu may meet many more patients who are quite open about their religious orientation than will the therapist working in private practice in a Northeastern metropolis. I work in a small university town in central Michigan. Though this area is largely rural and fairly conservative, my patients tend to be more sophisticated and better educated. However, if the patient is the first of his family to attend college, then religious issues are more likely to emerge. The patients I work with typically do not bring religious issues into therapy initially nor do such issues *appear* central to their difficulties, though in fact, at times such issues are crucial. Thus, I prefer to allow these issues to emerge in the same way as any other issues in treatment. This leads to a corrollary position. The presence or absence of a religious orientation in a patient only becomes a therapeutic issue when the patient's difficulties with others or his internal conflicts are expressed in a religious idiom. Religious expression is a medium which mirrors the quality and pattern of the patient's object relations (Rizzuto, 1979), and can also serve as a resistance to therapy. As well, the patient's personal religious configuration is an idiom that reflects, in part, those developmental events that have deeply challenged the patient's adaptive capacities, and which contains clues to significant past interpersonal experiences (Stolorow & Atwood, 1979). My own thinking about my patients stems basically from an ego psychological, object relations point of view. Religious material that appears in therapy and seems related to resistance or ongoing dynamic issues is handled in this context.

Religion gives organization and meaning to the world, and thus the patient's particular religious system tells a great deal about the patient's experiences and symbols. However, psychotherapy is an alternative way to give meaning to the world and can be used in ways which appear to compete with religion. This competition is sharpest when the patient's religious attitudes and practices are pervaded by those characteristics psychotherapy is most likely to effect. The therapist needs to exercise appropriate caution in interpreting the personal, dynamic roots of particular religious symbols. On the other hand, challenges may come unexpectedly and some risk-taking may be required.

THEMES: SOME OPENING ISSUES

The issues discussed here are not the only ones that will appear in therapy with religious patients. Many of the typical issues are illustrated by the case of Mr. A. described below, but I believe these issues are common to therapy in general. For example, there is the matter of interpreting religious terms and lables. A patient may ask the therapist "Are you a Christian?" or "Have you been saved?" at the very outset of therapy. In the context of a very conservative, evangelical, or fundamentalist ("fundamentalist" has become a disparaging term and many now prefer to use conservative or evangelical, though some will use fundamentalist proudly) position, this question may lead to miscommunication. A therapist who is, perhaps, Methodist, Lutheran, or Catholic, may respond that he or she is indeed a Christian but this response means something quite different for the questioner who is really asking whether the therapist has accepted Jesus as his or her personal savior, and perhaps has been baptized in the Holy Spirit. The latter is a specialized religious experience much more common to Holiness and Pentecostal churches.

Mr. A., whose case is more fully discussed later, came from a strong Lutheran background and sought relief from persistant hallucinations. He was hounded by divine and devilish themes and preoccupations which appeared frequently in his hallucinations. Fairly early in therapy he expressed his impression that I was an atheist. When I replied that I was Jewish he appeared relieved to know that, although I was not Lutheran, I at least espoused some religion. While it is common for therapists to inquire into the patient's motives for asking personal questions, religious patients will likely experience this as evasive so my practice is to give at least a limited answer and then explore how they feel about my response or what it means to them.

More discreet, tactful, or sophisticated patients may be more subtle than Mr. A. which gives more opportunity for therapeutic exploration. Yet the religious issues that lay below the surface and do not overtly signal their problematic character can be more troublesome. For example, Mrs. B. referred herself because her third marriage was failing and she had begun to suspect this had something to do with her. During the first interviews, she disclosed that her father had been a fundamentalist Baptist minister for many years. Later in the first session, I inquired as to how she had come to see me. She indicated that she had taken some psychology courses and had been impressed with behavior modification, though she did not think this was needed for her kind of problem. She was in the midst of a course in personality theory which she found interesting. At the end of the session, she added that she just did not buy the idea of "children lust-ing after their parents." Since she had identified herself as the daughter of a minister, I assumed that she must have been drawn into church services and other church-related activities and had received strong religious messages about the expression of proper behaviors and correct beliefs (this was later confirmed). I replied that there was nothing in therapy she had to believe except what she was convinced of out of her own experience. She then entered therapy rather willingly and dealt successfully with much traumatic material. In this instance, an initial communication with potential relevance for a religiously-oriented patient was addressed without any direct reference to religious values on either the patient's or the therapist's part.

The reverse can also occur. Frankly religious material may actually refer to quite different matters. Mrs. C. was a young woman active in her church's devotional and social activities. In her first therapy session, she expressed frankly several religious doubts. While some of her friends and associates would discuss "the gifts of the Spirit" and had no trouble believing in the literal inerrancy of the Bible, Mrs. C. wanted to discuss social issues such as world peace. She admired those who were certain the Bible was inerrant, but she had some reservations. The matters she presented in the first session would certainly sound like religious issues had I not known that she was a member of a tolerant, mainline Protestant denomination, relatively untroubled by theological rigor and purity. Had she come from a Pentecostal, Holiness, or conservative Baptist church, these issues would have had a quite different character. Instead, the issues she presented turned out to relate more to general personal doubts and insecurities expressed in a religious idiom than to deeply troubling religious-theological issues.

INTIMACY

Problems of intimacy are ubiquitous in therapy of both religious and non-religious patients. However, those patients, such as Mrs. B., who grew up in homes saturated with religious values and practices tend to be particularly wary of too great an emotional investment in therapy and the therapist. This was also seen in the case of Mrs. D., a woman in her late 30's, who was referred becuase of her

confusion and distress over having inexplicably caused the collapse
of her apparently satisfactory marriage. She received a strict Catholic upbringing, had gone to parochial school until she went to college, and had always been a dutiful child and adult. During the
course of therapy she become aware of my interest in religious issues
through her friendship with a colleague. After about a year of
therapy, we began to explore in much detail the complementary aspects of intimacy and autonomy in her life. She became aware of affectionate feelings toward me as sessions were increased to twice a
week. She oscillated between affectionate and frightened reactions
from session to session and this culminated in her lending me (at my
request) an old pamphlet related to her parochial school experience.
Her fears of therapy came more sharply into focus as she expressed
indirectly the idea that being close to me or to anyone seemed to
mean having to adopt their values. He fears had now intensified,
and she was essentially demanding an explanation of what was going
on in therapy, what were we doing; i.e., what was I *doing* to her?. I
tried, initially without much success, to explore what she felt was
happening to her. I assured her that I did not want to take her over,
but wanted to help her understand herself. Though there was no immediate reaction, subsequent sessions yielded increased clarity on
her dependency wishes and there was tentative emergence of some
aggressive impulses. While her fears of my control were not directly
interpreted, the patient very soon connected these fears to specific
elements of her prior Catholic upbringing, and particularly to an
overly close, though innocent adolescent relationship with a priest.

GUILT, GUILT FEELINGS, AND RESPONSIBILITY

Therapists and theologians use the very important concept of
guilt quite differently. This can lead to troublesome and mostly unnecessary misunderstandings on the everyday pastoral-therapeutic
level. In Christian theological terms, sin involves alienation from
God, while guilt is the objective emotional state that derives from
this basic situation. Guilt in the religious sense is usually attached to
a variety of failures on a behavioral and doctrinal belief level. In the
specific practice/belief system of the individual patient or denomina-

tion, guilt can take many forms.

When therapists talk of guilt or guilt feelings they are referring to something rather different. In general usage, guilt feelings include regret and self-criticism over having done something which would be regarded as wrong within most value systems. For therapeutic purposes, guilt feelings tend to be viewed more often as attached to events that are displaced from their original sources, or are a defense against feelings of helplessness, or a way to suppress angry impulses directed at someone, and so on. Therapists might refer to this as neurotic guilt while theologically, guilt is an objective, factual condition based on alienation from God and does not necessarily connote the therapeutic concepts mentioned above.

Theologically, if one bears guilt, one has the responsibility to make amends through repentance and reparation. From a psychodynamic point of view, such responsibility requires the capacity to be relatively free of unconsciously motivated repetitions and transferences. This leads the therapist to take a generally neutral stance with regard to feelings and behavior in order to expose unconscious material so that it may be bought within the control of the ego and worked through. Yet religious patients may not accept the need for this work and may resist efforts to modify or interpret infantile or ritualized modes of repentance or guilt-reduction. Further, they may avoid the exploration of deeper motivations of an apparently religious preoccupation with guilt and repentance. Communication can be impeded between therapists and patients who lend different meanings to the concept of guilt. This is illustrated in the following case.

Mr. E. married very early after graduation from high school and much before he was ready. Later, in the midst of advanced professional study for the law, marital difficulties surfaced and he entered therapy. During this time, he was unable to sustain the marital relationship, so he left his wife and two children to live with a younger woman. Despite intense feelings of guilt about the relationship with this younger woman, which were bolstered by parochial education in grade and high school, he was unable to extricate himself from this attachment. His guilt feelings arose both from the obvious pain his wife was experiencing through his rejection of her as well as the strict religious values inculcated by his home and his religious schooling. Therapy was bogged down due to various guilt-motivated resistances. Since therapeutic exploration and interpretation did not resolve the situation, I commented during one session that he seemed to need to "finish" his adolescence. This helped reduce his paralyzing guilt and therapy began to go forward again. Eventually, he and his wife were able to restore their marriage.

As we approached termination, the patient reviewed his therapy. In discussing this particular session, he rather blandly remarked that it had been a good growth experience for him and that it aided his marriage and his children. In a considerable departure from neutrality, I replied "Bullshit! What are you telling me? You abandoned them, you left them in the lurch!" His smile disappeared and he much more soberly agreed that he had, and that he could see the effects on his children. I suggested that he had work to do with them, and left it at that. During the termination phase, Mr. E. was attempting to come to terms with his prior religious rearing. Both his religious and familial upbringing emphasized belief based on faith and were experienced as controlling and intrusive. Now he was in a secular field (law) that emphasized and valued rationality. Rationality had become a defense against his deeper, conflictual feelings. I had, in a sense, given him permission to act out what he was going to do in any event, through the rationalization of his needing to "finish" his adolescence. It therefore seemed that I should be the one to correct through this later, blunt intervention the superego lacunae I had inadvertently reinforced.

CASE ILLUSTRATION: MR. A.

The case to be presented here will be described much as the material unfolded to give a sense of the therapy as it occured. Some material not central to religious issues will also be given to allow a better grasp of the overall case.

Mr. A., age 27, was referred to me by a colleague in Mr. A.'s home city some 50 miles away. Mr. A. had been discharged from the military on psychiatric grounds, had spent some time in psychiatric wards both before and after his discharge, and had been unsuccessfully treated medically for several years prior to coming to me.

During this period, Mr. A. received VA disability benefits and worked inconsistently. He presented himself to me as having tried all sorts of medication and now wanted "psychoanalysis" since medication had not helped. Due to bureaucratic delays, diagnostic testing could not be arranged until way too far into therapy. Overall, Mr. A.'s combination of strengths and weaknesses suggested a diagnosis of borderline functioning on a low level. I offered him psychotherapy on a once weekly basis (partly because of transportation constraints) and he agreed.

Mr. A. entered the military at 18 following an unhappy childhood and adolescence. He was the second of six male children and the older four were each two years apart. The two youngest were still in public school while the older three siblings were all apparently functioning successfully in diverse careers. Mr. A.'s father was a physician and his mother a nurse. The father appeared to be the dominant force in the family and had a history of alcohol abuse and extra-marital affairs. His role as the mother's instrument for physical punishment of the children was only divulged much later. Mr. A. felt that he never could win his father's approval and recalled a history of recurrent derogation and intrusion from the father. The parents were in the process of divorce and the mother was going to raise the youngest two boys herself.

When Mr. A. entered the service, he undertook strenuous training in an airborne, emergency medical evacuation program. He was apparently doing well for several months but as he neared the end of the program, he experienced increasing stress until, from his description, he had some sort of transient psychotic reaction involving visual and auditory hallucinations, accompanied by the fear of danger. He was hospitalized in the military psychiatric facility and once attempted to strangle a non-commissioned officer. After a stint in this psychiatric unit, he was discharged home where he attempted suicide. Over the next couple of years, Mr. A. was in different VA facilities and at least one private hospital. Thereafter he slowly improved over a period of three years, moved away from home to a moderate size city where, at the age of 24, he married a young woman 18 years old. A year and one half later he began therapy as the birth of his first child was approaching. At the time, he had no income other than VA disability benefits.

In our second session together, I showed Mr. A. the letter I had
written to the VA describing my clinical assessment of him and re-
questing that therapy be approved for payment. Mr. A. had investigated the situation beforehand and found that benefits were
available. He asked a question about a technical term in the letter
("ego-alien") which I explained. He then commented that he had always wanted to know what they wrote about him on "the psych
ward" but they would never tell him. This led into a discussion about
his father who, as I had suggested in the letter, figured significantly
in Mr. A.'s choice of a medically-related military speciality. He asked
for an explanation of his hallucinations which I explained as
thoughts projected onto the outside world.

Mr. A. then raised the topic of religion. He had experienced conflicting messages. His father was a hell-raiser and drinker, giving the
impression that religious values did not count for much, while his
mother was active in the Lutheran church. He wanted to know
where I stood. I did not respond specifically but assured him that I
considered religion important and then sought to explore his views.
Many sessions later he told me he thought this was typical professional evasiveness. We ended with Mr. A. saying that either his, or
the world's problems go a long way back. The next two sessions introduced most of the remaining themes that would arise over the
next one and a half years of therapy. In the first of these sessions, he
reported that his wife gave birth, and talked of his relations with his
in-laws which were better and more satisfying than with his own
parents. He reported several repetitive hallucinations: a voice called
him "Oops", which led to his feeling that he was a "mistake", and he
saw a visual hallucination of a series of stars that went, with a clicking sound, into a hole in the heavens covered with a rainbow.

In the next session, he described his efforts to get support from
Vocational Rehabilitation to return to school, and described working
both in his backyard and refinishing furniture. He talked of his need
to be perfect, which I interpreted to him as an antidote for low self-
esteem. The connection to religious themes of perfection in Christianity was not yet touched upon since the patient has not raised
such issues directly, and this was early in therapy with a patient distrustful of professionals, such as his father. He recalled a memory as
a very young child at home upstairs behind a baby gate and hearing

the washing machine making noise and thinking that it was going to get him (probably a screen memory). He also reported early feelings of being alone and feeling that the world was merely a figment of his imagination. He described more about his "breakdown" and how, after one of his hospitalizations he was discharged aburptly and called his parents. His father came and picked him up and he felt a great calm, as if God had come, and his symptoms disappeared for the next 10 days or so. The symptoms then began to return and it was at this point that he made a serious suicide attempt.

In the next session, he gave me the following note which is reproduced below without corrections.

DR. I ENVY THE PEACE OF MIND YOU MUST HAVE. I WISH MY UNIVERSE WAS NEAT AND TIDY WITH NO GAPING HOLES IN IT. ONE PART OF MY MIND LOOKES AT THE REST OF MY MIND WITH A COLD CRITICAL OUTLOOK, AND THIS THING I SEE SEEM TO SAY TO ME THAT MY PRAYERS ARE EMPTY AND THERE IS NO GOD. I HAVE A CONTANT STRUGGLE TO GO TO SLEEP EACH NIGHT, AND I HAVE TO TAKE MEDICINE TO DULL MYSELF TO INSENSETIVITY TIME(10:25)

What appeared to be a developing idealization was not interpreted at this time.

While this summary of the case material may make it seem relatively orderly and systematic, the experience in the therapy did not emerge as clearly. Mr. A.'s wariness and at times disorganizing anxiety as we touched painful topics, and his confused sense of reality when he was hallucinating, all complicated this beginning phase. Mr. A.'s father was clearly a significant figure, yet his mother's absence was conspicuous in the associations produced during sessions. The early memory of the dangerous washing machine and the sense of being alone in the world suggested early abandonment, while the material about the mother using the father to administer punishment at the end of the day came much later and confirmed this picture. I felt that interpretations about the father could be safely introduced as the material emerged, but that too much inquiry about the mother would further erode his already shaky attachments and seemed risky unless he was already clearly in touch with some directly hurtful act.

The following two sessions were further developments of the prior material. He reported that he had dreamed and, although he did not remember the dream, his wife had heard him talking in his sleep. According to her account, Mr. A. dreamed that he was on a building and saying, "It'll take six of you to throw me off this building, sucker, and I don't even see four of you." He did not have associations, but there were several dynamic configurations of four in his family; he is one of four brothers close in age, and his three brothers in this group plus his mother (or father) make a foursome. There are similar configurations of six so his parents are also implicated. There emerges, then, a general feeling of being different from and threatened by members of his family. More self-critical material emerged in the session, including a recent incident where the parents were having a fight, and he physically intervened. He prevented his father from hitting him and felt guilt for having shamed his father as well as guilt for wanting to hurt him. I first inquired into Mr. A.'s behavior in some detail, and then reinforced his self-restraint. I firmly distinguished between his feelings and his actions but did not touch the oedipal theme.

Mr. A. forgot his next appointment. I called him and he came. In that session it quickly developed that he was beginning to fear the relationship, overtly because the VA was not yet paying the bill and he was afraid of what I would want from him instead. In the same session, this was confirmed by his recalling that when he was 11 or 12, he ran away from home one night in the middle of winter because his father reprimanded him for not doing the dishes while the father was out earning a living. He continued on about his hallucination of a devilish image which he felt I would not understand or accept because I was an atheist. When I replied I was Jewish, he felt much relieved and recalled how he regarded my initial statement about religion in the second session, that "religion was important," as the usual professional evasiveness. I commented that we could be different and still work together. He appeared to accept this and we went into further exploration of the hallucinations. This led to his feeling that they were from the Devil and they went far back in his mind. I strongly interpreted these as feelings stemming from mistreatment as a child and this seemed to relieve him a bit.

Religiously-related themes diminished for a while in therapy and, as we concentrated more on the nature of his relation with his father, there was some preliminary reduction of his hallucinations and a diminution of anxiety. Early in the next group of sessions he described an incident at the age of 11 or 12 when his father directed him to kill a cat in the barn which he reluctantly did. He heard kittens mewing and when he told his father, he was forced to kill them too. I responded to this by saying that it was a very unkind thing for the father to do to a child and at this point he gave me the following letter. The letter is reproduced without corrections but this time the letter was written in cursive script rather than the immature block-lettering of the previous letter.

> This is how I see what you say. This man (my dad) has great power over me, or had, he influenced my character so much that I must confront the "enemy" and work things out. I have hurt so much, some unconscious some conscious, that I would just asoon let it "ride" in the sense that I still love and respect my father for what he is *inside* him down deep, than dwell on how outside influences have changed him into something that I dislike and even maybe hate. I realize my father is human like me, and he won't admit he was wrong about certain things to me. It seems he has constructed his own false universe to give him peace of mind while he is alive. God be with him then, I am not the Judge, God is! Maybe he had no Idea he had influenced my feelings so much, Im sure he didn't. I think he tryed to help me avoid problems that he had, and in doing so expected me to be just like him.

Mr. A. continued to come regularly and, on his own, also reduced his use of the major tranquilizer he had been prescribed. A dream at this time of vomiting his medication was interpreted as his feeling he had been given "bad medicine" in the hospitals. He confirmed this and discussed more openly his feelings about his experiences with military psychiatry, the V.A. psychiatric hospitalizations, and the various civilian psychiatrists he had seen. Reports about the military were most confused because he was in an acute episode then, but he was much clearer about subsequent experiences and had little of a positive nature to say. He was also taking sensible actions to protect and increase his benefits.

Mr. A.'s fear of being controlled by the treatment, which at the same time he regarded as helpful, continued to emerge as did more hallucinatory experiences of being watched, especially when he did poorly, or thought he did poorly at some activity. The emotional impact of his father's intrusions and control was more fully explored as Mr. A. reported how his father used to say "I know all about you" or "I can read you like a book". He had powerful *déjà vu* experiences which were not easy to clarify, but these, coupled with prior hallucinatory experiences of buildings melting, were interpreted as related to his father changing the rules on him and being omniscient. Much more anger emerged toward his father and doctors in general. He was able to say that the thing that watched him was God (a temporary shift in the quality of this image). I was able to connect this idea to the experience of his father as like a god when he picked up Mr. A. after his discharge from one of his hospitalizations. Connecting this "thing" that watched him with his father who, as a doctor and father was like a god to him, was followed by more intense anger to doctors. This anger was intensified by a series of unpleasant experiences with psychiatrists both during and after his hospitalizations, but he was also aware of his feelings toward his father. He disclosed that he, too, felt like a god during his "breakdown".

His troubled and painful identification with his father through the idiom of religious imagery was coming into sharper focus, though its meanings and dimensions were not fully clear to me. Though the religious imagery was clearly an important idiom for the expression of his conflicts, it was only pursued as it came up in therapy and I took care not to express special interest in it. His relief that I was not an "atheist" was not a resolution of his apparently "religious" concerns. His immediate acceptance of me as a Jew and not an atheist seemed only a way to preserve me as a partly good object. Too much interest in his religiosity appeared to risk arousing his fears of my wanting to convert him or to attack his faith. Since some Lutheran churches may still use hymnals containing prayers for the conversion of the Jews and he was deeply attached to the Lutheran church, I anticipated that he might fear conversion by me.

In the thirteen sessions between March and the end of June, Mr. A. regularly atteneded his appointments except for two times when he lacked money for gas and once when his wife gave birth. The next fifteen sessions from July until my vacation the week before Christmas were marked by slowly increasing difficulty in coming to his appointments, increasing difficulties with his wife, intensification of stress, and hallucinations. This phase began with two significant dreams. In one, he was being pursued by police and he fled into a cave which turned out to be a garage. Accompanied by two male companions (probably his brothers nearest in age with whom he was closest), he was followed by three bats (the police). He took the keys from a one-seat red sports car, but a middle aged, heavy-set woman said she had called the police so he gave her the keys and left. In the second dream he got a call from both his mother and father who sounded happy. His associations indicated the bats were connected to his father's common use of the expression "a bat out of hell". The red of the car was probably also connected with hell. He had just gotten a car from his mother which he had not yet paid for. The woman in the dream resembled his mother in hair color and looked like a woman who lived downstairs who was very abusive to her son but appeared superficially nice to others. His interest in getting something from a woman (cars in dreams are often body symbols) risked his father's disapproval. The wish for the parents to reconcile (in part to protect him from his oedipal impulses) seems clear in retrospect, although the session was much more confused because of his anxiety. Interpreting the mother's probable abuse seemed premature while we were still dealing with Mr. A.'s father. Splitting the mother and father images into kindly and painful affects was probably in effect, but not yet interpretable. I did not regard the oedipal material as central because his problems were rooted much earlier, having to do with fears of abandonment, annihilation, and external control.

Right after this session, Mr. A. was notified that, based on an extensive report I had submitted on him, his application for Social Security Disability was approved. In the next three sessions, his problems with his wife intensified. She was unhappy with being tied down with a young baby and also felt he was not giving her enough time and attention. In the last session before my vacation in August, he reported a hallucinated image of a face watching him when he and his wife were having intercourse. This face was the same critical face that watched when he was doing poorly and which most likely derived from an introjection of the father's criticisms. Both the earlier dream of the police and now the appearance of this face during intercourse were clearly oedipal. I missed this point at the time because of theoretical assumptions about the etiology of his difficulties. This was a significant blunder. Instead I supported his reported effort to have a different quality of marital relationship than did his parents (he helped around the house, did some housework).

When therapy resumed in the Fall, Mr. A. brought his wife to the first session because of their marital troubles (I had made this option available to him). Her transferences from her father to him were gently pointed out in terms of her expectation that Mr. A. would be as steady and persistant in projects around the house as her father was. Her father was also disabled for many years, but neither this, nor her desire to be a mother very early (she was 19), was commented upon. After this session, further arguments with his wife led Mr. A. to have a brief sexual encounter with another woman, but he did not have the experience of the hallucinated face. At this point, the oedipal material was explored and interpreted. I indicated that he was afraid of his father if he was to be a male and compete for his mother's attention, and that his wife appeared more similar to his mother after their child was born. Further, I suggested that his fear of being a successful man would be experienced as a dangerous accomplishment. The interpretation seemed to make an impact on Mr. A. This was followed by a week free of the use of medication until he and his wife had further conflict.

Mr. A. was increasingly more able to explore his hallucinations, though they were still very frightening. We spent time understanding his cosmic hallucination of a series of stars (points of light) that went clicking, one by one, into a rainbow. Earlier his associations to the rainbow were of something soft and pretty (and probably related to his mother). The stars or sparks were related to an ether-sniffing incident with his younger brother who was experimenting with fruit flies. After some ether inhalation, Mr. A. woke up grabbing at the flies and they reminded him of the sparks. Associations to masturbation led to a link between fruit flies, sparks, and sperm. During sex, he felt a loss of something, and when he hallucinated the sparks, a voice would be heard saying "there goes another one" or "you lost another one." Shortly after this session, he called about 5:30 A.M. to tell me of his idea of a new approach to physics which had to do with space, atomic particles, and gravity which was somehow connected to the Father, Son and Holy Ghost. While I had trouble following the content of his theory, I did not directly oppose it or try to interpret it. I suspected that he was beginning to feel more anger, now more directly aimed at me, and this was interpreted. In the past couple of weeks he had voluntarily made some payments on his bill from the accumulated Social Security Disability benefits (the V.A. was still mired in bureaucratic red tape), and after the previous payments there had been a call in the middle of the night. His payments were made in face of increased pressure from his wife regarding money.

This was followed by increasing pressure from his hallucinations and his recall of a dream at age two or so of an angel touching him on his behind with a wand that had a star on the end. As well, he had inserted marbles in his anus and it felt good, but he felt it was wrong. At about 10 his older brother initiated sexual intercourse with him and it tickled. He also talked of his father having an office downstairs. I suggested that he sought his father's love any way he could, even if it meant adopting a homosexual position. I interpreted his anger at his father as first being internalized but was now projected onto Satan and as coming at him from the devil. I said Satan comes from *sahtan* (adversary, in Hebrew) and is not a real person. These were his feelings, too.

The following session he told of having figured out the meaning of one of the names his voices call him: "Igglebop." This meant stupid or dummy, but also seemed to mean "wiggle Bob" (Bob is his father's name). He was still concerned with how the universe could change like it did. Before his breakdown, he believed the brand name of his parent's refrigerator was Amanda, but afterwards it was Amana. He associated Amanda to a witch's name. When I made the connection to his mother, he felt that I had somehow changed and that there was something there behind me. Whatever it was, it was a great mistake, he felt. I took this as a warning not to go further on the issue of his mother at this time. He then went on to say that his father, who had begun to have affairs six months after his parents were married, had gotten his mother pregnant again so she would not leave. This birth was probably Mr. A. and I pointed out how he must have felt he was a "mistake" in someone's eyes. Earlier in

therapy I had wondered how he knew much of the material he reported, and what now emerged was that the parents' private affairs
were well known in the family through the efforts of the mother to
gain allies. I later also found out that his father disclosed a lot to Mr.
A. Mr. A.'s distrust and suspiciousness were intensified in the next
session which he spent discussing his new theory of physics. The
stress he was feeling, plus continued money difficulties, led to a
month's interruption in therapy. There were phone contacts during
this time and one session was done by telephone because of his
financial problems.

We resumed therapy after Christmas and this new six month period was marked by fairly steady and more solid improvement as
well as a diminution of issues related to religion. In spite of Mr. A.'s
wariness, he was able to talk about his distrust of me, his mother's
use of his father to punish the children, and his strong fear that the
expression of his anger would lead to punishment and rejection, as
he felt it had in his family. His self-punitive superego was interpreted
as an attempt to make his unconditionally bad situation at home
conditionally bad — if the troubles at home were his fault then they
could possibly be corrected. These interpretations were made with
much more firmness and began to have an observeable impact. He
was beginning to recognize that his father's rejection of him arose
from the father's problems. This formulation later had to be modi-
fied as it became clearer that his father was in fact more intensely involved with Mr. A. than with the other siblings. Material then
emerged which showed that the father had shared with Mr. A. a
good deal about his own adolescent difficulties, including the father's
revulsion toward homosexuality and his early determination never
to let others hurt him. Mr. A.'s troubled identification with, and attachment to his father was becoming clearer. All this material was
summarized for Mr. A. as indications of the father's problems. I haz-
arded an interpretation that the father must have been the second
child or second son in his own family or origin as was Mr. A. and
that Mr. A. was the garbage pail for the disposal of the father's own
negative self-image. When Mr. A.'s recollections confirmed this pre-
diction, his negative self-image began to weaken. At the same time,
he began to feel that I really was concerned for him. His hallucinatory voice was now saying "You're *not* Igglebop." This stage initiated

an increase in Mr. A.'s objectivity and understanding.

While the hallucinatory experiences again began to decline in intensity, Mr. A.'s difficulties with his wife increased. After two months in a distant city on a job which temporarily interrupted therapy, they returned to the area. Joint sessions were arranged, and their communication patterns were examined. Mrs. A. wanted her husband to know what she needed without her having to tell him. Discussion helped her see this as unreasonable and she agreed to accept a referral for therapy. Their ways of circumventing each other were identified; he by presenting her with a *fait accompli* and she by withholding her thoughts. My availability re-aroused his fears of homosexuality, and I told him people could like each other without their relationship having to be sexual. This led to greater comfort in the session for Mr. A.

Although we will return to religious issues in the discussion section, it may be noted here that Mr. A.'s religious imagery was determined by problems at several developmental levels. The devilish face that watched and criticized him, along with the critical voices, seemed primarily related to oedipal difficulties. The senses of danger he felt also indicated the persistence of earlier fears of annihilation, pointing to difficulties in the first year (Blanck & Blanck, 1974). The rainbow hallucination was more obviously connected to Mr. A.'s mother, but this devouring image retained a positive valence for much of the course of therapy and was never fully explored because of his inability to tolerate the inquiry. It seemed to me that his initial religious exposure gave him some measure of contact with a fantasied good mother, through his mother's involvement in the Lutheran church. His aggressive, dependent, and sexual impulses were externalized through the devilish image through this image also punished him for these wishes. In fact, after leaving therapy he became involved in a conservative church which elaborated his cosmic imagery through the Book of Revelations — and which, I believe, temporarily stabilized him. He was able to utilize his new religious affiliation to identify with Jesus as his Saviour and thus join with the only beloved Son of a divine, but distant and painful Father. This paralleled his life situation rather well.

As we entered the second half of the year, Mr. A. still reported hallucinations, though these continued to recede and he was able to recognize the voice tone as similar to, if not identical with that of his father. This recognition further reduced the stress he felt. His difficulties with appropriate expression of anger was a recurrent theme thoughout this time. The religious overtones of these issues were expressed in forms similar to the following.

Mr. A. would occasionally bring up biblical injunctions to not be angry and to love others. My approach was to direct him to read the "love your neighbor" statement in Leviticus 19 with attention to the context of this injunction. I suggested that what was being emphasized in the Bible was loving assertiveness, rather than total suppression of one's angry feelings. At that time, I also interpreted his need to be a failure both as a way to meet his father's unconscious messages as well as to weaken himself so as to prevent him from discharging his anger. This enabled the therapeutic relationship to become somewhat closer and more mellow. This was also followed by an intense eruption of anger as he felt his problems were worse. What eventually emerged was passive, anal homosexual fantasies, and in the next session (the last before my summer vacation) he sat as far away from me as possible and asked if I were the devil. The intensity of the session and the patient's premature departure that day precluded sufficient exploration and interpretation of the meaning of these developments at that time.

In an emergency session Mr. A. requested during my summer vacation, he expressed his wish for a Christian therapist and I indicated that I had no wish to take him over nor did I wish to take away the good things he had gotten from his parents. He then brought up an experience that occurred six months earlier when I had supported his efforts to find a full-time job and he felt something from me going into him. Connecting this with his most recent fears of me, I again repeated that a positive relationship between two men does not have to be homosexual although I did not interpret his wishes for such a relationship at this point.

The fall was the concluding period of the active phase of therapy as Mr. A. eventually found a job in a distant city that paid a living wage. During this time the hallucinations had declined and were now experienced more like feelings. A crucial event then occured that solidified the correctness of some of my interpretations for the patient. He had telephoned his father who rejected him during their conversation. Crying while he was talking to his father, he also found himself smiling and feeling pleased. He could now appreciate the degree to which he had internalized the need to be a failure, and felt more able to tolerate his father's rejecting behavior.

Early in this period, Mr. A. discussed his mother in one session and his thinking became noticeably looser. Again this topic had to be deferred. More time was spent in joint sessions with Mr. A. and his wife helping them improve their communications. Her efforts to control her husband were interpreted with little effect and since they were soon to be moving, hopefully to continue in therapy, the matter was not pressed. After they moved, there were several calls. Mrs. A. called to complain about her husband and I tried to direct her back to working out communication with him and continuing in therapy. Mr. A. called at one point and informed me that his hallucinations were back. I replied by asking who had said something nice to him the day before, since we had clearly identified his need to be a failure in order to win his father's love. This question startled him, and he recalled that it was the foreman. This produced a dramatic disappearance of symptoms. Mr. and Mrs. A. became involved in a local church that seemed to be pentecostal and evangelical. He became deeply involved in religious activities, particularly focused on the Book of Revelations and the person of Jesus. As noted above, this may have helped him to feel an identification with a loved son. Several months later, I received partial payment, along with the following letter.

Dear Bob,

Shalom — hope you and your family are blessed. I have been praying for you every night (almost). I have been praying that you have a memory lapse and forget I owe you $700.00. Seriously though I am grateful for what God has done you for me. Have you ever read Matt 24:32-34 Jesus is saying that when israel (Blossoms) the generation that sees this won't pass but all profecy given about the end of the world comes to pass. Any way that's enough Bible lesson. O, one more, according to Genesis man didn't eat meat until after the flood (Genesis) Write me a letter

Take care

Tom

This was far from a finished therapy and the stability of Mr. A.'s gains depended on his continuing in therapy when we stopped.

DISCUSSION: COUNTERTRANSFERENCE

As a Jew transplanted from New York to a small Midwestern town, I am sensitive to being a member of a minority group exposed to conversion attempts. Jews have been subject to conversion attempts of varying degrees of cruelty and contempt, and certain forms of Christianity contain a strong strain of hatred and attempted rejection of its Jewish parentage (Ruether, 1974). I believe I was thus particularly able to empathize with Mr. A.'s fears of conversion although his fears had a specifically Christian background. From the latter stages of therapy on, I found several of Mr. A.'s efforts to convert me irritating at times, though I recognized he felt he was giving me a great gift. Though the person wishing to offer conversion to me may mean well, it is at the expense of my personal heritage and some form of denigration is implicit. Professionally, I attempt to be receptive to what the patient is trying to say but, if the matter is pushed, I have to make clear what the boundaries are. The patient will then experience feelings of rejection and these have to be dealt with within the therapeutic context.

At times Mr. A. wanted my agreement with or acceptance of certain matters, such as his theory of physics, which were of obvious importance to him. Maintaining a neutral stance without his feeling rejected required careful navigation, especially since this theory was confused and did not make sense to me. On the whole, I feel that the greater portion of my discomfort was not specifically related to religious issues, but to working with a very troubled man who lived 50 miles away, and without a reliable psychiatric backup for medication and psychiatric paperwork, except for a nine months period. Further, his unreliable car, his wife's fears over and interference with the therapeutic relationship, and the fact that the V.A. lost the original paperwork leading to a delay in payment, added to the difficulties. The primary source of countertransference was the intensity of the material he would produce and its confusing and rather direct primary process aspects.

RELIGIOUS ISSUES

There is generally good therapeutic reason for therapists to not be too self-disclosing, particlarly at the start of therapy. With more disturbed patients, some flexibility is justified. In this case, it probably would have been useful to freely indicate that I was Jewish when Mr. A. raised the question during the second session. The question of whether the patient and therapist should share the same religious background is less significant in my view provided the therapist does not make assumptions about the patient's background and is willing to learn about it. Mr. A. spoke of wanting a Christian therapist at one point. It was crucial at that time to recognize this request as not only presenting a religious issue but a dynamic one: it served Mr. A. as a much needed defense against his homosexual impulses. And so it seemed more useful to deal with his latent fears of control and intimacy than to treat his request on the surface level of our religious congruity, though this might have been a realistic issue at certain other phrases in therapy.

One of the central issues in this case is the way in which Mr. A.'s use of religious and cosmic imagery expressed significant developmental experiences and an impoverished quality of his object representations (Stolorow & Atwood, 1979). At the beginning, Mr. A.'s alienation from any good objects, his punitive superego, the empty, punctured quality of his world, and his general psychological pain were plainly conveyed in his first note to me. God was "good" perhaps, but also distant and cold — and all the while devilish images pursued him. The division seen here may have been a splitting defense, supported by conventional religious imagery. For a long time there was a clear separation between his "bad" father and "good" mother. Early on he held to the idea that there were some good things about his father in spite of the generally negative picture, but exploration of negative aspects of his mother remained intolerable. His ability to actively seek help, to deal rationally with mundane problems with his VA benefits, and to pursue education while still struggling with his hallucinations, indicated that he had indeed internalized some good qualities of his father and that splitting may not have been the primary defense. The cosmic rainbow which swallowed points of light was for a long time also viewed positively, but later acquired an evil tinge in his hallucinations. His symbolisms might have been different had he been Catholic, in which case he might have had conveniently available a mother figure in Mary (Oetting, 1964), but the degree of object relational impairment would presumably have been similar. The devilish image that watched him seemed to be an introject of the critical, largely oedipal father who would punish him for his wishes toward his mother. As the father's real qualities were explored and interpreted, the devil largely disappeared from his life as did most of the other hallucinations. Dealing with the homosexual fears also helped relieve his psychotic symptoms, but his homosexual wishes remained largely unresolved at the time therapy stopped.

When Mr. A. moved out of the area to find a job, he carried through his effort to continue therapy. His increasing religious interests led him to find a Christian counselor, but the therapy did not go on for long, in part because of problems with V.A. benefit payments. He became very involved with a pentecostal type of church which emphasized the Book of Revelations and speaking in tongues. He was also "saved," which meant taking Jesus as his pesonal savior. This suggested dynamically that he identified with the only beloved Son of a divine Father and this may have provided a supportive resolution for his conflicts, although his intense enthusiasm led to occasional complaining calls from his wife who was not as enthusiastically involved with this church. The Book of Revelations is a very difficult document, full of intense, obscure imagery of an apocalyptic nature. His attraction to this imagery appeared consistent with his prior hallucinatory experiences of buildings melting, evil forces, and cosmic (heavenly) signs, such as the rainbow. This was not an altogether encouraging development, however, and suggested a considerable reservoir or unresolved issues.

While religious issues wove a thread through much of Mr. A.'s therapy, these were rarely dealt with in isolation from the ongoing treatment issues. I once commented that Satan was not an actual person but a Hebrew word for adversary, leading to the interpretation that Mr. A. had devilish feelings which he externalized onto a concrete concept of a Satan. Another time, in dealing with anger, I suggested he read the full section on "love your neighbor," but I was not then sufficiently conversant with relevant New Testament materials which would have added weight to the intervention. It is easy to enter into discussions of religious issues in therapy but, as a Jewish therapist with a Christian patient, this is risky early in therapy as it is likely to be seen as an effort at conversion which would be experienced as pressure on already shaky ego boundaries.

SUMMARY

The therapist who is interested in and responsive to religious issues in therapy can become overinvolved or relatively underinvolved in them, to the detriment of the ongoing therapeutic work. Unlike some (Ellis, 1970, 1980; Fromm-Reichmann, 1950), I think religious issues often can be very important. This material may provide clues to object relations, and identifications, and may even support resistances, but such material is not the primary vehicle of therapy. Rather, the therapist needs to be prepared to meet religious material with knowledge and respect while attempting to advance therapy as best he or she can. While the pentecostal churches and the practice of glossolalia are not patterns of living that personally appeal to me at all, I thought it a workable solution for Mr. A. at that point in his development. To be able to feel loved by Jesus represented a much improved set of object representations for him. Other issues remained. He might have stayed for further therapy had his wife been more supportive. I did not feel in a position to deal very effectively with her undermining of Mr. A.'s investment in therapy of her need for him to be "sick." To a degree, she was his only good relationship. Once she entered her own therapy, I felt reluctant to interpret her undermining even though it had become clearer to me by then. When the A. family moved to a distant city, she did become involved in his church activities so there were further possibilities to work out both their personal and marital problems.

REFERENCES

Adams, J. E. *Competent to Counsel*. Nutley, N.J.: Presbyterian and Reformed Publishing Co., 1970.

Atwood, G. The loss of a loved parent and the origin of salvation fantasies. *Psychotherapy: Theory, Research and Practice*, 1974, *11*, 256-258.

Beit-Hallahmi, B. Encountering orthodox religion in psychotherapy. *Psychotherapy: Theory, Research and Practice*, 1975, *12*, 357-359.

Balnck, G., & Blanck, R. *Ego psychology: Theory and practice*. New York: Columbia University Press, 1974.

Coyle, F. A., Jr., & Erdberg, P. A liberalizing aproach to maladaptive fundamentalist hyperreligiosity. *Psychotherapy: Theory, Research and practice*, 1969, *6*, 140-142.

Ellis, A. The case against religion. *Mensa Journal*, 1970, *138*, 2-4.

Ellis, A. Untitled paper presented at a symposium on Religion and Psychotherapy at the American Psychological Association Convention, Toronto, 1978.

Ellis, A. Psychotherapy and atheistic values: A response to A.E. Bergin's "Psychotherapy and religious values." *Journal of Consulting and Clinical psychology*, 1980, *48*, 635-639.

Evans, H. S. The Seventh-Day Adventist faith and psychotherapy. In R.H. Cox (Ed.), *Religious Systems and Psychotherapy*. pp. 89-97, Springfield, Il.: Charles C Thomas, 1973.

Fromm-Reichmann, F. *Principles of Intensive Psychotherapy*. Chicago: University of Chicago Press, 1950.

Gersten, L. The mental health needs of the pious. *Sh'ma*, 1979, *167*, 52-55.

Kagan, H. E., & Zucker, A. H. Treatment of a "corrupted" family by a rabbi and psychiatrist. *Journal of Religion and Health*, 1970, *9*, 22-34.

Lovinger, R. J. *Working with Religious Issues in Dynamic Therapy*. New York: Jason Aronson, (in press).

Oates, W. E. The diagnostic use of the bible. *Pastoral Psychology*, 1950, *1*(9), 43-46.

Oetting, E. R. The treatment of interpersonal relationships in psychotherapy as a function of religious socialization. *Journal for the Scientific Study of Religion*, 1964, *4*, 100-101.

Pruyser, P. Assessment of the patient's religious attitudes in the psychiatric case study. *Bulletin of the Menninger Clinic*, 1971, *35*, 272-291.

Pruyser, P. The seamy side of the current religious beliefs. *Bulletin of the Menninger Clinic*, 1977, *41*, 329-348.

Ragan, C., Malony, H. N., & Beit-Hallahmi, B. Psychologists and religion: Professional factors and personal belief. *Review of Religious Research*, 1980, *21*, 208-217.

Rizzuto, A-M. *The Birth of the Living God: A Psychoanalytic Study*. Chicago: University of Chicago press, 1979.

Ruether, R. R. *Faith and Fratricide: The Theological Roots of Anti-Semitism*. New York: The Seabury Press, 1974.

Spero, M. H. Countertransference in religious therapists of religious patients. *American Journal of Psychotherapy*, 1981, *35*, 565-575.

Stolorow, R. D., & Atwood, G. E. *Faces in a Cloud*. New York: Jason Aronson, 1979.

Vayhinger, J. M. Protestantism (Conservative-Evangelical) and the therapist. In R.H. Cox (Ed.), *Religious systems and Psychotherapy.* pp. 56-71. Springfield, Il.: Charles C Thomas, 1973.

Chapter 10

RELIGIOUS CONVERSION AND PARANOID STATES AS ISSUES IN THE PSYCHOTHERAPEUTIC PROCESS

LEON SALZMAN, M.D.

THE presence of religious issues in mental disorders deserves special emphasis because of the frequency and intensity with which the two mesh and because of the unique role religious feelings and beliefs play in human development and functioning. Psychotherapy of the emotional disorders must concern itself with the role of religious phenomena as potentially both a constructive as well as destructive force. While religious feelings and practice can promote the development of moral standards and ethical values which support stable and healthy personality integration, religiosity can also be used as a delusional structure to support a weak ego and give an illusion of strength and integrity in a disorganized personality.

In the therapeutic process one must distinguish between these qualities and functions, and differentiate delusional from valid or mature ideology. One does not merely assume that diverse or alien religious attributes or behavior are necessarily pathological. On the other hand, the therapist must recognize the metaphoric use of religious terms and avoid theological dispute or disagreement. Religious conversion is one instance of the potential use of religion as a defense tactic, or as a metaphor for distress, dissatisfaction with, or threat to one's functioning as a healthy individual. In several studies on religious conversion and faith healing, I have documented both aspects of the religious concerns. Techniques for handling the patient's religious ideas are therefore closely related to the function such ideas serve in the person's life and his neurosis or psychosis.

SPURIOUS VERSUS TRUE RELIGIOSITY

Mysticism, fanaticism, stigmatization, asceticism, flagellation, scrupulosity, and conversion must be viewed in psychological and spiritual terms in order to differentiate true or constructive religious expression as opposed to exploitative or spurious religiosity. I make this distinction not so muct on the basis of the orthodoxy of persons' beliefs vis-a-vis some normative religious definition as on the basis of the social and intrapersonal consequences of the religion for the particular believer. From this point of view, "spurious religiosity" could be characterized as negation rather than affirmation and as estrangement from reality and one's fellow man, while "true religiosity" is a positive affirmation oriented toward objective reality and one's fellow man in a constructive, benevolent, and affirmative sense.

What I refer to as spurious religiosity was described by Nietzsche as an effort to reach a higher world by casting off this one. Nietzche pointed out that the ascetic personality is probably satisfied personally but keeps concealed from the world his lust, pride, and feelings of superiority. He aims to fly beyond the ordinary human. Others describe spurious religion as that which offers temporary consolation by aiding the devotee to avoid struggle instead of facing and fighting it out, as in movements such as anti-alcoholism, theosophy, technology, palmistry, nudism, etc.

In evaluating true versus spurious religiosity, it is important to include in the assessment all aspects of the individual's activity in addition to his professed spiritual beliefs. Phenomena which the individual in earlier years considered to be of divine origin may now be recognized as derived from discoverable physical causes, and vice versa. As the individual moves through the various stages and subphases of psychosexual, psychosocial, and self-development, transformations occur in the quality of religious experience and the content of religious imagery and so forth — all of which merit careful consideration.

The problem of religious conversion is of great interest in this regard. Religious conversion is a specific instance of the general principle of change in the process of human adaptation. In the process of fulfilling human needs, some people follow a rather direct course with minimal strife and turmoil, while others face major obstacles which require deep-reaching adjustments. These major adjustments may constitute constructive, forward-looking change or they may result in regressive movements.

Most and possibly all change is gradual in its development, but since it culminates in a specific moment of ideological alteration or conversion may seem to the observer to be an instantaneous, unexplained, mysterious event. However, in every case there has been an incubation or preparation, with lesser or greater struggle, and then a final triggering or precipitating event or confluence of events which produces the apparently sudden, dramatic, and obvious change. Where a profound change in philosophy, ideology, or ethics occurs, the hidden but encompassing struggle is particularly significant. Thus conversion cannot be regarded as a sudden or dramatic event although under extremely hazardous and life endangering circumstances profound changes may occur with only limited background and preparation. I consider conversion to be any change of religion or of moral, political, ethical, or aesthetic views which occur in the life of a person, with or without a mystical experience, which is motivated by strong pressures within the person. The conversion experience as I define it is not necessarily identical with "religious experience," although this may sometimes result in conversion. Religious experiences, which may be defined in an infinite number of ways, seem frequently to involve cosmic feelings, states of rapture and mystical phenomena, and can be likened to the "ecstatic absorption" occurring when a dissociated tendency reaches awareness and threatens the integration of the personality. In some personalities these experiences are followed by intensely creative and rich religious and psychic growth, while in others such experiences may initiate or exacerbate schizophrenic process. (It is worthwhile to note that psychological insight, such as during therapy, often occurs along with profound feelings of expansion, a sense of cosmic identification, and so on, which resemble elements of the religious experience.)

DEFINITIONS OF CONVERSION

James' (1902) work remains one of the best descriptions of the process of conversion. James views conversion as a struggle away from sin rather than as a striving toward righteousness. He considered it an attempt to handle the problems of dispair, anger, worry, and fear; after becoming exhausted with the struggle and giving up, the person deals with these feelings by adopting opposite feelings. Conversion is thus depicted as a passive rather than active process; a self-surrender to achieve unification in which personal will must be given up; an uncontrolled eruption of unconscious needs into consciousness. James thus describes all conversion similar to the way I describe regressive conversion since it occurs within the framework of severe emotional stress and anxiety and is an attempt to deal with pressing psychological problems.

In 1928, Freud wrote a short essay on religious conversion in response to a letter from an American doctor describing his conversion experience. The conversion had occurred following an intense emotional experience in the morgue when the doctor, then an intern, saw a "sweet old lady" on a slab. In analyzing this experience, Freud noted that the conversion occurred following intense reactivation of early odeipal hatred of his father. This hatred succumbed to a powerful opposing current and ended in complete submission to the father in the form of Christ. In his short paper, Freud touched on an important dynamic process involved in conversion and uncovered one of the core elements of the conversion process although he did not document it in further writings.

Usually it appears to have been sufficient that the person proclaimed his newfound faith. The theologians have generally not been concerned with the impetus or motivation, provided the proclamation of faith conformed to their concept of the religious doctrine. Moreover, reports of mystical phenomena accompanying conversion experiences have tended to make it more acceptable to theologians.

TYPES OF RELIGIOUS CONVERSION

In a general sense there are two major types of conversion:

1. *Progressive or Maturational Conversion.* This type frequently occurs in the course of real maturing. It takes place when after a reasoned, thoughtful search the person adopts new values and goals which he was determined to be higher than those he has abandoned. It occurs in reasonably normal persons, and when it is *religious* conversion, represents the achievement of the ultimate in the humanistic religions; it expresses the positive fulfillment of one's powers with self-awareness, concern for others, personal integration, and oneness with the world. It may, of course, be a political or ethical conversion or it may be a spiritual conversion quite outside the framework of conventional religion. I call such conversions progressive, but only in the sense that the movement is forward in terms of personality development, permitting greater maturity. These progressive conversions usually take place largely on a conscious level. The struggle involved usually concerns the dynamics of love as opposed to "care," and represents the person's endeavor to expand and to express his creative, positive, kindly attitudes toward his fellow man and the world at large.

2. *Regressive or Psychopathological Conversion,* which is illustrated in this chapter. Theologians have stated that "man's extremity is God's opportunity." This appears particularly applicable to regressive conversion, for it tends to be a highly charged, profound, emotional experience which occurs during attempts to solve pressing and serious problems in living, or to deal with extreme disintegrating conflicts. It may take the form of a mystical emotional change in religious affiliation or a sudden, dramatic surge of enthusiasm within the framework of the individual's own group. The qualities of religiosity *and* personality typically seen in such conversion mark it as a pseudo-solution, likely to occur in neurotic, prepsychotic or psychotic persons, although it may also occur in presumably normal people when they are faced with major conflicts or insuperable difficulties. Thus, while regressive conversion is often considered an abnormal, even psychotic de-

velopment, this is not necessarily the case. However, because it is brought out by increasing anxieties and has a disjunctive effect on the personality, it may either precipitate or be part of a psychotic process. At the same time, because the conversion experience itself may include some conjunctive elements, and because of its defensive nature, it may ward off incipient psychosis.

I designate regressive conversion only in the sense that such conversion produces changes which for the most part are defensive solutions and partake of the characteristics of psychopathological phenomena. While the motivations and conflicts may appear similar to those in the progressive conversions, the dynamics of regressive conversions deal with affects other than love and the outcome is manifestly different.

CASE 1: MR. A.

Mr. A., raised as a devout Protestant, converted to Catholicism at age 18. He consulted me when he was 46 years-old for help in dealing with his impotence and with an overwhelming compulsion to make a scene in church by screaming obscene words at the priest. His difficulties with his compulsive behaviors during church services forced him to sit in the aisle seat of the last row, so he could escape quickly when he felt impelled to shout insulting, lewd, and obscene remarks.

The patient reported that at the time of his conversion he had been involved in a powerful struggle with a hated, alcoholic father whom the patient believed was cruel to his mother. He remembered that his prarents were locked in endless, bitter conflict. As a child, the patient was extremely attached to his mother and was her confidante, which seriously impaired his developing sympathies with his father. The mother would regularly describe the father's sexual behavior in vivid detail to the patient, probably in order to fortify her son's attachment to her, and unconsciously to encourage the seductive, incestuous liason between her and the son and act out her hostility to her husband. On one occasion when the patient was 15 years-old, he almost killed his father after his mother told him of a perverted act his father had committed upon her.

During his adolescence, the patient was a participant in choir in his church, in the course of which he met a minister who made homosexual advances to him. The sexual stimulation which probably stirred up his own latent homosexual orientation precipitated a transient psychotic episode during which time he had delusions about being Christ and other religious figures. These served as a defense against any greater awareness of his homosexual trends. At this time he converted to Catholicism and spent a brief time in a psychiatric hospital. Following his discharge, he attempted to enter a monastery, but was refused admission. Shortly after this he married and in the following years began drinking heavily. Six years before he elected therapy with me, he consulted another psychiatrist for impotency and on the latter's recommendation he received testosterone treatment. He benefitted only to the extent that the psychiatrist became his friend and idealized father-figure.

The patient consulted me following the death of this psychiatrist. He seemed extremely shy and displayed a surface friendliness. He initially expressed devout interest in the Catholic Church and emphasized its value to him. He deplored his wife's lack of interest. She has half-East Indian and had been brought up as a Catholic in a convent, but disliked what she considered the Church's hypocrisy. Beneath his superficially amiable attitude the patient was hateful; his attitude toward everyone was prejudiced, cynical, sarcastic, and deprecating. He hated his "half-breed" wife who did not come up to his expectations. His formerly great affection for his mother had slowly turned into hatred as he came to feel she had emasculated him by her constant descriptions of his father's various perverse acts towards her. He now visited her only infrequently because of the fierce, almost unrestrainable destructive feelings he had toward her. He felt superior, critical, and contemptuous toward me because I was Jewish. He viewed my Jewishness in stereotyped ways, describing me as aggressive, materialistic, and pushy. He was distressed by my authority and prestige, which he intimated was undeserved, since I had not hailed the new Savior. He hated his boss and his brothers, and despite his expressed devotion to the Catholic Church and his faithful attendance and attention to all religious forms such as Communion, he was also critical of the Church's doctrine of original sin and man's essential evil. Through the patient's morass of hate one could feel his yearnings for peace and closeness. His extreme loneliness prompted constant drinking. At the same time, his sensitive longing for a more spiritual existence and his wish to deal productively with his many intense hates were reflected in his lifelong interest in music and now in psychotherapy.

In the course of our work it became clear that his conversion to Catholicism occurred at a time when he was overcome with intense feelings of hatred toward his father and toward the minister *cum* father-figure who had made homosexual advances to him. The temptations induced by these advances mobilized a violent, explosive anger within him which, in turn, resulted in conversion partially as an attempt to be relieved and expiated by God. While the conversion did not forestall his subsequent paranoid schizophrenic illness, the clinical evidence suggested that it had reduced its potential severity — his hospital stay was short and there had been no recurrence of psychotic symptoms afterwards. But his overwhelming hate remained, pervading his whole existence.

In the course of psychoanalytic work, the patient's hatred towards his father disappeared. In clarifying his transference, he could acknowledge that his contempt for me was unjustified and based on his resentment toward his father and the priest who attempted to seduce him. Authority meant therapist, father, priest, and the dogma of Catholicism. In recognizing and experiencing his identification with the aggressor, in this instance priest and authority (Church), he had attempted to resolve conflict by conversion and being a super-devout, scrupulous believer. On a number of occasions we constrasted his hateful, bitter, vindictive attitudes with his professed religious attitude of love and forgiveness. He was slowly able to acknowledge that his conversion was a defense against his extreme hostility rather than an affirmation of love and devotion. These insights helped him understand his compulsive obscenity in Church as the escape of repressed hostility and oedipal rage. As we explored his relationship with his mother and his wife, it became abaundantly clear that he shared his mother's antagonistic views because of the security and power it afforded him in his early years. He was eventually able to understand that his mother's views of his father were based on her own neurotic needs, and he began to see his father in a new light. He developed instead a nostalgic attachment for him, feeling especially sympathetic toward his father's creative and artistic interests. We recognized that religious concepts and ideas served primarily as cloaks for his confused sexual identity, and his resentment and hatred of his parents, and his efforts to resolve his homosexual inclination. Since the last conflict was stirred up by a priest this conflict was expressed in religious terms and an attempt at solution was framed in religious ideology and dogma.

Mr. A saw the male as a supreme, idealized authority, identified in the priest (religious power) and in the intense anxiety stirred up by the attempted seduction. This trauma renewed his extreme hostility toward men which could be restrained only by a reaction-formation of becoming the devoted, dedicated discipline-son. In his metaphor, this meant becoming a dedicated religious figure. Often he would quote Scriptures to avoid confrontation of his anger, and I would insist that he look at his own behavior rather than the virtues of Christ and Christianity. At other times he would attack my lack of religious conviction in order to mitigate my observations of his use of religion as a distracting element in our relationship.

At all times I refused to discuss theological issues, insisting that our concern was his psychological self; namely, how he dealt with anxiety in interpersonal relationships, rather than the existential anxiety of ultimate concerns and meanings. At such times, he would accuse me of being an atheist and unworthy of his regard. We would then reexamine the purpose and motivation of his accusations to discover the tranferential elements as well as the tactics for displacing his anxieties onto others. Thus religious doctrine and ideology was recognized as defensive techniques to avoid acknowledging his own anger and to distance any male or authority figure, lest he experience closeness or tenderness. At times when he would be grateful and experience some closeness to me he would discover and express some new criticism of my lack of understanding or religious feelings. On one occasion he was thankful when I made a time change for his convenience and he was able to acknowledge his embarrassed uneasiness when I pointed it out to him. This was the beginning of much insight into this paradoxical behavior in dealing with tender feelings.

We avoided issues of dogma and dealt instead with his use of religious metaphor as a defense against his extreme feelings of anger and his profound need for love, acceptance, and intimacy. Mr. A. became aware of his fondness and regard for his father in nonsexual terms. Finally, he was able to come to terms with his heterosexual adjustment and related more tenderly toward females; namely, his wife and mother. His is presently working through his relationship with his mother. The patient's present understanding of his religious conversion is that it was an incident occurring in the "aggressive, neurotic course of my life." Although he is still Catholic in form and attends Church regularly, he continues to be beset by theological doubts and could not be described as following a fully religious life. He remains actively hateful of the Protestant Church and is intolerant of all other religious groups. However, as he experiences more tenderness and permits more intimacies, he will undoubtedly alter much of his hostilities to other religious groups and moderate the scrupulosity in his Catholic observance. His religious feelings will become more true, valid, and less defensive, and the extremes of devotion will no longer be required as a defense against doubts and dangers.

CASE 2: MR. B.

Mr. B. converted to Catholicism at age 22, following years of religious indecision. His problems included a suspicious, hostile attitude toward the world, especially toward the Catholic Church. The patient's history included a running battle with his father which continued up to the father's death, in which the patient was indirectly involved. His father, who was a tall man, was rigid and autocratic. He favored his first-born son, who was taller and more worldly than the patient. Mr. B. was short statured and physically weak and felt despised by his father. His academic success in school failed to win his father's respect and Mr. B. increased his rebellious and antagonistic activity in an effort to force some kind of recognition from his father. The mother was a weak, impotent, midly-accepting figure in the family who dedicated her life trying to make peace between Mr. B. and his father. Her place in the patient's life seemed to have been comparatively unimportant.

Mr. B.'s father followed the forms of the family religion, but his attitude toward it was contemptuous and he was without real values or ethics. Mr. B. was more idealistic and was troubled by his father's hypocrisy. For a while he conscientiously attempted to conform to the ethics of the family's religion, but the atmosphere of his family made this impossible.

The estrangement between the patient and his father continued to widen, and their reltionship was finally ruptured by Mr. B.'s conversion to Catholicism. The conversion, which Mr. B. had contemplated for along time, took place after a girlfriend of his own faith rejected him. In part, the positive aspects of the conversion grew out of a warm friendship with a priest who assumed a foster-father role toward the patient. Several years after joining the Church the patient married a Catholic girl.

The patient's hatred of his father, while less extreme and less manifest than Mr. A.'s, has been relentless and thus far insoluble. His attachment to the Church appeared to be more pure and spiritually-based than in the first case, but it was also characterized by constant quarrels with priests and by a covertly hostile attitude. As these issues emerged in our work we separated his hostility towards his father from the metaphorical "father" as exemplified in his religion and the priesthood.

By way of illustration of one aspect of our work, during several sessions the patient inadvertently spoke of Father (priest) when he meant father (biological). While this might be considered common among Catholics, it generally does not occur so deeply involved with resentments and hostilities as it did in Mr. B.'s case. He also saw the Church as an unfriendly, demanding, repressive force, symbolized by his priest, and almost an exact replica of his family life. During these sessions he was amazed to discover that he confused "priest" and "father" in his thinking and feeling. This insight played a major role in elucidating his confusion and eventually resolving it.

CASE 3: MISS C. AND HER MOTHER

The third case concerns the mother of a patient, Miss C. The mother's psychopathology so definitely contributed to Miss C.'s becoming a paranoid schizophrenic. The mother despised her husband

and never wanted any children. However, after 2 years of marriage she became pregnant. After the birth of her daughter she gained 100 pounds, which she blamed on her husband and continually berated him, accusing him of having ruined her life. She communicated this feeling to her daughter, who regarded her father as a helpless, stupid dolt.

When Miss C. was 8 or 9 years-old, her mother had a conversion experience, and with revivalistic furore left the moderate Protestant sect to which she belonged to join a pentacostal sect. The conversion included numerous hallucinatory phenomena and the adoption of a most rigid, formalized dogma. Concerning her mother's conversion, the patient had spontaneously observed that it was "born and nurtured of hate and guilt." The patient consequently viewed religion, and particularly her mother's religiosity, as phony, deceitful, and an attempt to overcome her hatreds and unfilled life. During the course of understanding her mother's emotional difficulties and her resentments toward her father and men in general, Miss C. recognized that the conversion experience did reduce the extremity of her mother's despair and meaninglessness. The patient, however, was bitterly anti-religion, distrusting all men, authority, and the Church in particular. Religion, for her, conveyed neither love, trust, nor acceptance. It was a ritualistic, super-moralistic attack on other denominations and religious orientations other than one's own.

A feeling of rivalry with an intense hatred of men, as conveyed to the patient by the mother, lay at the core of Miss C.'s paranoid problem. In this case, our therapy involved dealing with her unsatisfied longings for a satisfactory heterosexual relationship. This longing was reversed and displaced onto the unworthiness and infidelity of males, and was denied by her paranoid suspiciousness and avoidance of them. At times this distrust was expressed in paranoid delusional terms. Repeated demonstration of this dynamic in many of her current experiences enabled her to abandon many of her paranoid and delusional attitudes toward men. Only when the patient's identification with her mother's neurotic abuse of religious attitudes was unfolded could the patient acknowledge her own distortions and prejudices toward religious feelings. These insights permitted her to distinguish between her mother's attempts at a religious solution for an intra- and inter-personal conflict and the mature healing value of

religious benefits and practices. These views were chrystalized when
we could demonstrate the differences in her mother's religious attitudes and those conveyed in the context of authentic religious teachings. This opened up for Miss C. a new world of the potentiality of
love rather than hate as a binding force in human relationships.

CASE 4: MR. D.

Another instance of the significance of religious symbolism and
ideology cloaking neurotic development occurred in a seminary student, Mr. D., who became violently delusional following exposure of
his homosexual tendencies in a bar near the French Quarter in New
Orleans. This episode followed an alcoholic spree after a seminary
examination period. While inebriated, Mr. D. provoked some
sailors at the bar who beat him up. He became delusional and spoke
of his stigmata, pointing to the fresh bruises on his hands and fore-
head. He insisted he personified the Second Coming and documented it by showing his bruises, claiming he was both Jewish and a
rabbi. A few days later, after repeated interviews and sedation, he
was able to identify that he had been beaten up by the sailors because he had tried to seduce them. He acknowledged this with hor-
ror and shortly thereafter resumed the delusion that he was the
Second Coming and that he was beaten because of his adventific
claims.

Mr. D.'s eventual awareness and willingness to entertain doubts
about the validity of his delusional claims enabled us to speculate
about the reasons for this delusional development. He reviewed his
earlier doubts about his masculinity and recalled earlier homosexual
episodes that he had completely repressed. He had hoped, in seeking
a religious life, to overcome these sexual tendencies and had
managed to abandon all sexual outlets until his drunken spree.
Upon initially recovering from his hangover with total amnesia of
the drunken brawl, he could not accept the real explanation for his
bruises, and dramatized them in religious terms with a grandiose delusional system. After repeated psychotherapeutic interviews and
the uncovering of many repressed feelings and events in his past life,
he could entertain the possibility that he had some homosexual in-

clinations which he was morally and psychologically unable to accept. Only after much exchange in encouraging him to accept the reality of his condition and to mitigate his moral detestation of homosexuality could he acknowledge the significance of his delusional system and his valid religious beliefs which he continued to honor and respect. At this point he was able to explore his grandiosity and its relationship to his suspicions and distrust of others. He maintained his religious convictions with more humility and true pastoral concern than he had before his psychotic episode.

CASE 5: MR. E.

Paranoid elaborations are frequent in delusional systems where religious claims or metaphors are used. In these instances the individual feels particularly victimized by the outbursts of those who jeer and disclaim the pretension of Christhood. An example of this occurred in a 35 year-old male, Mr. E. He was 26 years-old when he had his first paranoid breakdown as a student in a theological seminary. Prior to this he had been an energetic person, full of hypomanic schemes for the improvement of mankind and preoccupied with the superior, grandiose conception of his own abilities and capacities. He periodically got involved in large-scale adventures based on trivial ideas which he felt would be phenomenal if he could get the proper financial backing and so forth.

In one manic episode at the seminary, Mr. E. professed he was Christ, and then proceded to demand from his colleagues and the administraton the proper recognition for his "second coming." The paralogic for his delusion was interesting. It was based on the fact that he had some Jewish ancestry and that his mother's name was Maria. In addition, he was born outside New York, which is the capital of the world today, as Jerusalem is the capital of the Christian world. Like Christ, he felt no relatedness to his family. He saw himself as a truly universal man who had little of anything material and a great love for humanity. Most significant for Mr. E., however, was the fact that the Second Coming would be in the chape of an ordinary man who was unknown to the world. In his efforts to secure recognition for his divine self he antagonized the seminary adminis-

tration, became involved in extravagant dealings, passed some bad
checks, and was eventually hospitalized.

During this period of intense activity trying to establish his divinity, he developed many persecutory ideas, particularly that he was
being followed and, eventually, that his enemies were trying to kill
him. In a later episode, he attempted to kill his "persecutors," which
forced a second hospitalization. He was released from the hospital
when he denied his paranoid ideas and did not mention his belief in
his divinity. However, he continued to see himself as Christ until
only very recently, when the belief was finally questioned and abandoned.

What interests us here is the way in which his paranoid religious
ideas developed out of his grandiosity. At the outset he thought he
felt nothing but love and compassion for his fellow man and the wish
to fulfill his universal mission. Meeting with disbelief, antagonism,
fear, and distrust, he began to assume that there was an organized
attempt to deny him his proper role. Well-meaning friends and rela-
tives who attempted to tone down his claims were viewed as enemy
agents, trying to force him to relinquish his divinity. Neighbors and
strangers who accidentally approached him on the street or in other
public places were viewed as functioning by design and purpose.
Physicians, and eventually the police were enemy agents sent to confuse and destroy him. All this time he was confirming his divinity
through a rational though paranoid examination of his experience.
When doubts arose about the reality of his being Christ, he dealt
with them easily by insisting that he was not a true son of his
parents, but an adopted son, and that the difficulties in being recognized were further proof of the truth of his claims. This patient eventually socialized his behavior, refrained from mentioning his "true"
Christ identity, and functioned moderately well until he got involved
in more ambitious projects.

CASE 6: MISS F.

Miss F. came to treatment in a panic state following some fleeting
paranoid delusions. Her life was organized around being a dedicated missionary in the field of human relations. After a brief at-

tempt at reorganizing all of Christian education (!) and attempting to solve the world's racial problem, she became involved in a dynamically-oriented child therapy center, where she was forced to examine the premises of her behavior. This produced panic and fear of becoming insane, which led her to seek psychoanalytic treatment.

Our relationship developed in an atmosphere in which she would provide me with data about her superior, Christ-like devotion to human welfare. She hoped I would reinforce and reaffirm her notions in this regard. While she could acknowledge that something had gone wrong in her life she nevertheless expected to overcome these defects, through an insight or two and over a brief period of time, so that she could renew her salvation activities.

A typical picture unfolded during the course of early sessions. The patient was notably grandiose. She felt that her unique skills and understanding were constantly being hampered by stupid, contemptible people who were selfish and materialistic. She never examined the impact of her behavior on others and expected them automatically to acknowledge her good will even as she insulted them. She expected much more from the world than her position entitled. She behaved as though she were the only interested, honest, and unbiased worker, and could not understand why her activities, which people agreed with in principle, always produced such strong negative reactions. Her suspiciousness was conveyed in endless ways and ultimately in full-blown delusions about being followed, having her telephone tapped, and being the object of scrutiny by unseen security agents.

Miss. F.'s father was a prominent figure and public servant in a small western town. He was the leader in all "good" local causes. His self-righteousness was flavored with truisms and virtuous aphorisms, although he was indeed acknowledged for his good works in the community. Everyone, including his wife and children, viewed him as a holy, dedicated, and saintly person. It became apparent during therapy, however, that many of his noble projects were carried out at great emotional cost to his family. He was absent from home for long periods of time and deprived his family both financially and emotionally. The patient could win recognition and approval from him only by being his most active co-participant in projects of community interest and welfare. She was convinced early in life that only a selfless, dedicated program would satisfy her father. Being the best in her class was not satisfactory unless accompanied by an unselfish intention and scheme to aid mankind. Every need, interest, or activity needed to be framed in altruistic but actually unrealistic terms. She was required to be the most selfless Christian under all circumstances.

Miss F. had a brilliant academic career, becoming an acknowledged leader in college. Her relationships with her classmates were excellent though superficial, and she had many boyfriends with whom she developed idealistic relationships. While at college she had her first inkling of the extravagant nature of her goals. At this time she recognized that she would never be satisfied unless she became a figure of universal prominence and developed grandiose conceptions of her future.

After marriage she became involved in activities and organizations whose goals were the improvement of race relations and world peace. However, in some of these organizations she stirred up considerable antagonism and in other groups provoked outright attacks from colleagues. She was shortly rejected by other members of these organizations because of her fanatical zeal and self-righteous devotion. She then became a teacher, which eventuated in her psychotic episode.

Her activity in therapy paralleled and documented her difficulties in the outside world. She was markedly grandiose, always noble, honest, and dedicated. Her mission was to develop group relationships to ensure peace and good will. She planned to accomplish this through the message she had to deliver which she expected automatically to be received and accepted. She burked no exception or difference of opinion, and she never examined her behavior in terms of its effects on others since she assumed her views were beyond criticism or objection. Therefore, when there was some disagreement with her friends over a program of racial integration, her friends suddenly turned into persecutors who were tapping her telephone, having her followed and investigated, trying to disgrace her, etc. During the latter part of therapy, she said: "Most of my insecurities were handled by considering myself a great leader, a superman type of character. My behavior went along with this. I established a position as leader of a peer group and worked hard to maintain this position, often putting family responsibilities in the background in order to to this. I used the role of martyr to act out deep feelings of being unfairly treated and rejected . . . The idea of competition . . . the idea I am living with and working with people more mature and wiser than I am is impossible to digest even though I can cheerfully recognize such a situation."

Her relations with me mostly were that of a doting child who idealized her father and expected him to be all-knowing and perfect. This transference attitude prevented her from expressing openly her resentments and criticisms. However, she also was fearful of being abused and forcibly seduced by this overpowering authority who could injure her sexually as well as physically. She maintained this transferential attitude in spite of evidence both overt and covert, since I would frequently declare my realistic limitations and my own powerlessness. It was only as she developed more self-esteem and resolved her sexual ambivalence that she began to see me as a friendly, helping therapist and not a designing, exploitative man.

In pursuing her grandiose claims, she idealized a superman self-image and derogated all evidence of weakness and inadequacy in herself and others. She was contemptuous of the female, who signified the weak and ineffective member of society. In spite of a successful marriage and family and a satisfactory sexual adjustment, she attempted to deny the sterotypes of femininity such as dependency, weakness, and passivity. She frequently raised the question of her possible homosexuality and wondered how this could be since she idealized the male only for his status and had no sexual interest in the female.

In view of the importance of homosexuality in the development of paranoia, it is especially interesting to note that this patient presented no evidence of homosexuality, latent or manifest, conscious or unconscious, either in her wishes, fantasies, or dreams. Her orientation was feminine, including her resentment of the cultural privileges and prerogatives of the male, as well as envy of his strength and power. Her sexual orientation and interest could be conceptualized as "homosexual" only by strenuous forcing of the data to fit preconcieved ideas about paranoia. Her sexual activity was entirely satisfactory except when she felt she was being used only for sexual purposes. Although she responded actively and warmly to her husband's advances, she also searched for indications that he was primarily interested in sex activity and not in her as a person. When she enjoyed sexual contact the most, she resented it since sexual enjoyment implied to her that she was a wholesome female which in turn meant that she was weak and compliant as the stereotypes suggested.

In essence, Miss F. was confused and torn by her inability to form a clear sexual identity and role in her ambivalence and confusion about the gender stereotypes in psychological as well as social and philosophical theorizing. Thus, much of her behavior and attitudes were contradictory and disruptive to the pursuit of her life's goals and interests. So, too, was she torn between being a seductive female and an ascetic, dedicated mother, and daughter. The solution to this role confusion was to separate her real interests and desires from the jargon and psychological theories she was familiar with.

TREATMENT OF RELIGIOSITY IN PARANOID/GRANDIOSE PATIENTS

The maintenace of grandiose immunity from being human was necessary, as illustrated in Cases 3, 4, 5, and 6, to prevent what the patient feels will be the extreme opposite — that of utter helplessness and contemptuous failure. All standards, ideals, and activities were of extreme utopian order, which could not be compromised in the slightest. The patient demands automatic acceptance in order to avoid a realistic appraisal of his or her activities. Otherwise, they would have needed to confront the picture of imperfect humanness, leading to the destruction of the grandiose defense system and the reexperiencing of earlier childhood, narcissistic pain. In therapy, every budding awareness of imperfection was met by an immediate need to resolve the difficulty right now and for all time. The obvious incapacity to do this produced the outbreaks of anxiety, panic, and paranoid accusations.

The therapeutic skills necessary to deal with paranoid developments in patients require a thorough understanding of the adaptational value of such a defense. The paranoid process is designed to support an integration based on the notion of one's grandiose un-

iqueness, total independence, and omnipotent and omniscient capacities. This grandiosity stems from a deep sense of personal inadequacy and the danger of meaninglessness in accepting any
insignificant evidence of personal deficiency. Tenderness, closeness,
intimacy, or dependency is totally impossible since it indicates weakness and less than superhuman potentiality. The need for absolute
power and magical performance, divorced from realistic effort, ne-
cessitates total control over the environment.

The treatment of emotional disorders in which religious phenomena play distinctive roles requires skill in dealing with paranoid developments since they are frequently manifested in defenses. In
every instance it is an error for the psychotherapist to get involved in
theological discussions of dogma or ritual. However, it may be often
necessary to allow the patient to relate his religious background and
beliefs as they manifest themselves in the mental disorder. The
therapist's role remains that of investigating how he is treated or
used by the patient in the defensive elaboration of characterological
distortions, and reflecting this back to the patient, rather than to
take some moral stance on the validity of the patient's theological
concepts.

The resolution of paranoid distortions can only occur through a
direct confrontation of reality in an atmosphere already partially
open to confrontation. An illustration follows. I first saw Mr. L.
during a quiet period in his paranoid illness when he was unable to
go to work. He was being supported by his wife because he was offered no job worthy of his status. Besides, at any time the call might
come for him to acknowledge his "second coming," and he was holding himself ready for it. During the seven months I had been seeing
him, we attempted to reexamine his living with respect to the major
facets of his personality: his grandiosity, his contempt for the defi-
ciencies and weaknesses of others, and, particularly, his special significance as a multigenius who would eventually be acknowledged
and given his true reward.

During one interview he ruminated about a device he had
worked out to get larger rockets off the ground which would beat the
Russians and save our government millions of dollars. This lead to
much rumination about his brilliance and superman qualities and
ultimately his god-like qualities and perhaps being Chirst, himself.

We explored this and similar beliefs in the context of his arrogance and total lack of humility which were antithetic to the known qualities of Christ as humble and restrained. I pointed out numerous additional distinctions. While at first he was angered by what he considered my failure to acknowledge his genius and his accomplishments, he came slowly to agree that some of his "claims" were exceedingly unrealistic and grandiose. Gradually, he was able to understand his Christ delusion as the wish for total perfection in all things, and was eventually able to abandon this wish.

Certainly the issue is not finally resolved when an awareness, even as striking as this, occurs. It is only the beginning of therapy, with the way now open to investigate what necessitated the development of such a grandiose device to avoid humiliation and failure. It has long been felt that reason or logic cannot undo a delusion system. Yet we must consider this notion, since I believe it is precisely this approach which allows the paranoid to reexamine the premises of his delusion and, in accepting doubts about it, opens up the possibility of altering it. I am not referring to the naive notion that one can demonstrate through logical analysis or direct attack that the patient's delusion is impossible or that instruments such as he describes are non-existent (i.e., that he cannot be Christ since Christ is already dead). Such efforts are patently doomed to failure. However, the awareness that the paranoid delusion flows logically *from false premises developed by the patient's grandiosity* allows one to pursue the meaning and significance of the delusion as a logical consequence of conscious mentation. This is imperative in order to overcome the first major roadblock in the defensive structure of paranoid development.

The greater task in the therapeutic process is to enable the patient to experience satisfaction from real achievement in everyday tasks. Such success must be based on realistic performance and adventures and not from magical fulfillment of grandiose schemes. While it is difficult to encourage these patients to attempt what to them is a trivial enterprise, it often turns out to be highly gratifying. In this task, mature religious endeavors or involvements can be encouraged, monitored with the patient in the therapeutic session from a realistic viewpoint. Frequently it is their first true success based on a realistic appraisal of the challenges and their part in the solution of them. These people have often been rather successful, but they cannot appraise their productions since they are viewed in the light of their grandiose expectations. The grandiosity is a way of avoiding the tests of realistic performance and thus no real esteem is ever established. However, with the resolution of the paranoid and grandiose delusions, there is some chance for realistic goals to be set which these persons can achieve. It is these attainments which form the basis for prolonged remissions and ultimate recovery.

Therapy of delusional states which are distortions of conscious experiences must be dealt with in conscious, rational terms. In an atmosphere of tolerant yet obvious disagreement regarding the patient's misperceptions which arise out of them, the therapist must firmly and actively assist the patient in examining the multiplicity of possible interpretations of the patient's assumptions about the behavior of others. This can be done when some doubt is thrown on the validity of the patient's tubular orientation, opening up the arena for massive review. At this point we are allowed to investigate the source, aim, and dynamics of the grandiose processes in conventional psychotherapeutic fashion. This holds true when the delusions are expressed in religious terms in the form of scrupulosity, mystical identification with religious figures, or the assumption of being the agent of God, or God, himself. The therapist must first attempt to focus on the patient's potential doubts and uncertainties about these misidentifications before any further rational examination of them can take place. One does not boldly insist that the patient cannot be Moses, or Chirst, or that the excessive devotion or scrupulosity is irreligious. The attack must be sensitive and cautious in order to avoid immediate withdrawal and the accusation of being a partner to the conspiracies the patient has been fighting against. Discussions of dogma, religious concepts, and devotional rituals must be absolutely avoided in the face of strenuous efforts on the patient's part to embroil the therapist. One must always be on guard against the subtle and covert efforts to engage the therapist in theological arguments. If necessary, the religious counselor can be recommended for such discussions. Ultimately, the therapist must help the patient recognize that his religious concerns, as they ae reflected in his psychological problems, have a basis in anxiety, which, in turn, are based on concerns relating to his feelings of low esteem, unacceptability, feelings of being unloved, or incapable of being love, or whatever else is the source in that particular person. The focus in therapy is primarily the patient's anxieties and insecurities in other areas of his living. Once a trusting relationship is established, the therapist can then approach the delusion more directly, tying it to the patient's excessive needs for control and acceptance and demonstrating how the delusion is an attempt to achieve this power by a phantasied solution.

REFERENCES

Freud, S. A religious experience (1902). In *The Standard Edition of the Complete Works of Sigmund Freud.* vol. 21. London: Hogarth, 1958.
James, W. *Varieties of Religious Experience.* Modern Library, 1902.

BIBLIOGRAPHY OF SOURCES
DEALING WITH PSYCHOTHERAPY
OF RELIGIOUS PATIENTS

Allison, J. Adaptive regression and intensive religious experience. *Journal of Nerous and Mental Disease,* 1967, *145,* 952-963.

Allison, J. Religious conversion: Regressin and progression in an adolescent experience. *Journal for the Scientific Study of Religion,* 1969, *8,* 23-30.

Apolito, A. Psychoanalysis and religion. *American Journal of Psychoanalysis,* 1970, *30,* 115-123.

Atwood, G. E. On the origins and dynamics of messianic salvation fantasies. *International Review of Psychoanalysis,* 1978, *5,* 85-96.

Aviad, J. From protest to return: Contemporary teshuvah. *Jerusalem Quarterly,* 1980, *16,* 71-80.

Bergin, A. Psychotherapy and religious values. *Journal of Consulting and Clinial Psychology,* 1980, *48,* 96-98.

Berkower, L. Emotional problems of yeshivah students. *Tradition,* 1974, *14,* 80-89.

Bet-Hallahmi, B. Encountering orthodox religion in psychotherapy. *Psychotherapy,* 1975, *12,* 357-359.

Bet-Hallahmi, B., & Argyle, M. God as a father-projection: The theory and the evidence. *British Journal of Medical Psychology.* 1975, *48,* 71-75.

Boisen, A. *The exploration of the inner world: A study of mental disorder and religious experience.* New York: Harper & Row, 1952.

Bowers, M. K. *Conflicts of the clergy.* New York: T. Nelson, 1963.

Bronner, A. Psychotherapy with religious patients. *American Journal of Psychotherapy,* 1964, *18,* 475-487.

Bruder, E. Psychotherapy and some of its religious implications. *Journal of Pastoral Care,* 1952, *6,* 28-32.

Casey, R. P. The psychoanalytic study of religion. *Journal of Abnormal and Social Psychology,* 1938, *33,* 437-452.

Clark, R. Religious delusions among Jews. *American Journal of Psychotherapy,* 1980, *34,* 62071.

Cohen, R., & Smith, F. Socially reinforced obessing: Etiology of a disorder in a Christian Scientist. *Journal of Consulting and Clinical Psychology*, 1976, *44*, 142-144.

Cohen, R. Socially reinforced obsessing: A reply. *Journal of Consulting and Clinical Psychology*, 1977, *45*, 166-171.

Coyle, F. A., & Erdberg, P. A liberalizing approach to maladaptive fundamentalistic hyperreligiosity. *Psychotherapy*, 1969, *6*, 140-142.

Deutsch, A., & Miller, M. J. Conflict, character, and conversion: Study of a "new religion" member. *Adolescent Psychiatry*, 1979, *7*, 257-268.

Donschik, S. Some psychological aspects of the modern *ba'al teshuvah*. *Intercom*, 1979, *18*, 6-15.

Draper, E. Psychoanalysis and religion. IN R. H. Cox (ed.). *Religious systems and psychotherapy*. Springfield, Il.: Charles C Thomas, 1973.

Early, L., & Lifschutz, J. E. A case of stigmata. *Archives of General Psychiatry*, 1974, *30*, 197-200.

Ekstein, R. A clinical note on the therapeutic use of a quasi-religious experience. *Journal of the American Psychoanalytic Association*, 1956, *4*, 304-313.

Fauteux, A. "Good/bad" splitting in the religious experience. *American Journal of Psychoanalysis*, 1981, *41*, 261-267.

Frankl, V. *The doctor and the soul*. New York: Knopf, 1955.

Franzbalu, A. Distinctive functions of psychotherapy and pastoral counseling. *Archives of General Psychiatry*, 1960, *3*, 583-592.

Fromm, E. *Psychoanalysis and religion*. New Haven: Yale University Press, 1963.

Grant, V. Counseling for loss of faith. *Pastoral Psychology*, 1970, *21*, 22-30.

Greene, J. C. A "madman's" seraches for a less divided self. *Contemporary Psychoanalysis*, 1969, *6*, 58-75.

Guntrip, H. Religion inrelation to personal integration. *British Journal of Medical Psychology*, 1969, *42*, 323-333.

Halleck, S. Discussion of "socially reinforced obsessing." *Journal of Consulting and Clinical Psychology*, 1976, *44*, 146-147.

Kagan, H., & Zucker, A. h. Treatment of a "corrupted" family by a rabbi and psychiatrist. *Journal of Religion and Health*, 1970, *9*, 22-34.

Kiev, A. *Magic, faith, and healing*. New York: Free Press, 1964.

Knight, R. Practical and theoretical considerations in the analysis of a minister. *Psychoanalytic Review*, 1937, *24*, 350-364.

Krasner, B. Religious loyalties in clinical work. *Journal of Jewish Communal Service*, 1981-1982, *58*, 108-114.

Larsen, J. Dysfunction in the evangelical family: Treatment considerations. *Family Coordinator*, 1978, *27*, 261-267.

Levin, T., & Zegins, L. Adolescent identity crises and religious conversion. *British Journal of Medical Psychology*, 1974, *47*, 73-82.

Lewin, H. S. The use of religious elements in modern psychotherapy. *Journal of Pastoral Care*, 1950, *4*, 9-12.

Linn, L., & Schwartz, L. W. *Psychiatry and religious experience*. New York: Random House, 1958.

Littlewood, R. The antinomian hasid. *British Journal of Medical Psychology*, 1983, *56*, 67-78.

London, P. *The modes and morals of psychotherapy.* New York: Holt, Rinehart, & Winston, 1964.

London, P. Psychotherapy for religious neuroses? *Journal of Consulting and Clinical Psychology*, 1976, *44*, 145-147.

Lorand, S. Psycho-analytic treatment of religious devotees. *International Journal of Psychoanalysis*, 1962, *43*, 50-56.

Lovinger, R. Therapeutic strategies with "religious" resistances. *Psychotherapy*, 1979, *16*, 419-427.

Lubin, A. J. A boy's view of Jesus. *Psychoanalytic Study of the Child*, 1959, *14*, 155-168.

Mann, J. Clinical and therapeutic aspects of religious belief: A report. *Journal of the American Psychoanalytic Association*, 1964, *12*, 160-170.

Mann, K. W. Religous values and factors in counseling. *Journal of Consulting Psychology*, 1959, *6*, 259-262.

Meehl, P. Some technical and axiological problems in the therapeutic handling of religious and valuational material. *Journal of Consulting Psychology*, 1959, *6*, 254-259.

Mester, R., & Klein, H. The young Jewish revivalist: A therapist's dilemma. *British Journal of Medical Psychology*, 1981, *54*, 299-306.

Mowrer, O. H. (ed.). *Morality and mental health.* New York: McNally & Co., 1967.

Nadler, S. Torah-based family therapy. *Proceedings of the Associations of Orthodox Jewish Scientiests*, 1983, *7*, 51-70.

Nelson, M. O. The concept of God and feelings toward parents. *Journal of Individual Psychology*, 1971, *27*, 46-49.

Novey, S. Utilization of social institutions as a defense technique in the neuroses. *International Journal of Psychoanalysis*, 1957, *38*, 82-91.

Novey, S. Considerations on religioun in relation to psychoanalysis and psychotherapy. *Journal of Nervous and Mental Disease*, 1960, *130*, 315-324.

Oates, W. (ed.). *The religious care of the psychiatric patient.* Phila.: Westminster, 1978.

Oetting, E. R. The treatment of interpersonal relationships in psychotherapy as a function of religious socialization. *Journal for the Scientific Study of Religion* 1964, *4*, 100-102.

Ostrov, S. A family therapist's approach to working with orthodox Jewish clientele. *Journal of Jewish Communal Service*, 1976, *53*, 147-154.

Ostrov, S. Sex therapy with orthodox Jewish couples. *Journal of Sex and Marital Therapy*, 1978, *4*, 266-278.

Ostow, M. Transference and countertransference in pastoral care. *Journal of Pastoral Care*, 1965, *19*, 103-114.

Ostow, M. Social and psychological aspects of religion in psychotherapy. *Journal of Nervous and Mental Disease*, 1966, *141*, 586-594.

Ostow, M. The role of religion in psychotherapy. *International Psychiatry Clinics*, 1969, *5*, 77-92.

Pattison, E. M. Psychiatry and religion circa 1978. Part I. *Pastoral Psychology*,

1978, *27,* 8-25.

Pattison, E. M. Psychiatry and religion circa 1978. Part II. *Pastoral Psychology,* 1978, *27,* 119-141.

Pattison, E. M. (ed.) *Clinical psychiatry and religion.* Boston: Little, Brown, 1969.

Peteet, J. Issues in the treatment of religious patients. *American Journal of Psychotherapy,* 1981, *35,* 559-564.

Pruyser, P. Assessment of the psychiatric patient's religious attitudes in the psychiatric case study. *Bulletin of the Menninger Clinic,* 1971, *35,* 272-291.

Pruyser, P. The seamy side of current religious beliefs. *Bulletin of the Menninger Clinic,* 1977, *41,* 329-340.

Reissner, A. Religion and psychotherapy. *Journal of Individual Psychology,* 1957, *13,* 165-168.

Rizzuto, A.-M. Object relations and the formation of the image of God. *British Journal of Midical Psychology,* 1974, *47,* 83-99.

Rizzuto, A.-M. *The birth of the living God.* Chicago: University of Chicago Press, 1979.

Rizzuto, A.-M. Freud, God, and the devil and the theory of object representations. *International Review of Psychoanalysis,* 1976, *31,* 165-170.

Rizzuto, A.-M. The father and the child's representationof God. In S. Cath, A. Gurwitt, & J. M. Ross (ed.). *Father and child.* Boston: LIttle, Brown, 1982.

Rubins, J. Neurotic attitudes toward religion. *American Journal of Psychoanalysis,* 1955, *5,* 71-81.

Rubins, J. Religion, mental health, and psychoanalyst. *American Journal of Psychoanalysis,* 1970, *30,* 127-134.

Rutledge, A. Concepts of God among the emotinally upset. *Pastoral Psychology,* 1951, *2,* 22-27.

Salzman, L. The psychology of religious and ideological conversion. *Psychiatry,* 1953, *16,* 177-187.

Sevensky, R. Religion, psychology, and mental health. *American Journal of Psychotherapy,* 1984, *38,* 73-86.

Shands, H. Momentary diety and personal myth. *Semiotica,* 1970, *2,* 1-34.

Sharkey, P. W. (ed.). *Philosophy, religion, and psychotherapy.* University Press of America, Washington, D. C., 1982.

Slawson, P. Treatment of a clergyman: Anxiety neurosis in a celibate. *American Journal of Psychotherapy,* 1973, *27,* 52-60.

Smet, W. Religious experience in client-centered therapy. In M. G. Arnold & J. A. Garson (eds.). *The human person.* New York: Ronald Press, 1954.

Spero, M. H. Clinical aspects of religion as neurosis. *American Journal of Psychoanalysis,* 1976, *36,* 361-365.

Spero, M. H. Implications of countertransference for the religious therapist and client. *Journal of Psychology ad Judaism,* 1977, *1,* 36-51.

Spero, M. H. The contemporary penitent personality: Diagnostic, treatment, and some ethical considerations. *Journal of Psychology and Judaism,* 1980, *4,* 133-193.

Spero, M. H. Psychophysiological sequelae of holocaust trauma in a Jewish child. *American Journal of Psychoanalysis,* 1980, *40,* 53-66.

Spero, M. H. *Judaism and psychology: Halakhic perspectives.* New York: Ktav/Yeshiva University Press, 1981.

Spero, M. H. A clinical note on the therapeutic management of "religious" resistances in orthodox Jewish patients. *Journal of Jewish Communal Service,* 1981, *57,* 334-341.

Spero, M. H. The Jewish patient in psychotherapy: Diagnosis and treatment. In R. P. Bulka & M. H. Spero (eds.). *A psychology-Judaism reader.* Springfield, Il.: Charles C Thomas, 1982.

Spero, M. H. Countertransference in religious therapists of religious patients. *American Journal of Psychotherapy,* 1981, *35,* 565-575.

Spero, M. H. Psychotherapeutic procedures with religious cult devotees. *Journal of Nervous nd Mental Disease,* 1982, *170,* 332-344.

Spero, M. H. *Handbook of psychotherapy and Jewish ethics.* New York: Feldheim, 1984.

Spero, M. H. Religious patients in psychotherapy: Comments on Mester & Klein's "young Jewish revivalist." *British Journal of Medical Psychology,* 1983, *56,* 287-291.

Spero, M. H. A note on transference as a religious phenomenon. *Journal of Jewish Communal Service,* 1984, *60,* 183-187.

Spero, M. H. Theoretical and clinical aspects of transference as a religious phenomenon in psychotherapy. *Journal of Religion and Health,* 194.

Stamey, H. The "mad at God" syndrome. *American Journal of Psychotherapy,* 1971, *25,* 93-103.

Stark, R. Psychopathology and religious commitment. *Review of Religious Rsearch,* 1971, *12,* 165-175.

Stern, K. Some spiritual apsects of psychotherapy. In F. J. Braceland (ed.). *Faith, reason, and modern psychiatry.* New York: J. P. Kennedy, 1955.

von der Heydt, V. The treatment of Catholic priests. *Journal of Analytic Psychology,* 1970, *15,* 72-80.

Wagner, H. The adolescent and his religion. *Adolescence,* 1978, *13,* 349-364.

Wallace, A. The institutionalization of cathartic and control strategies in Iroquois religious psychotherapy. In M. K. Opler (ed.). *Culture and mental health.* New York: Macmillan, 1959.

Whitlock, F., & Haynes, J. V. Religious stigmatization: an historical and psychophysiological study. *Psychological Medicine,* 1978, *8,* 185-202.

Wikler, M. Fine-tuning: diagnostic techniques used by orthodox Jewish patients. *Journal of Psychology and Judaism,* 1979, *3,* 184-194.

Woollcott, P. The psychiatric patient's religion. *Journal of Religion and Health,* 1962, *1,* 337-349.

Woollcott, P. Pathological process in religion, In E. M. Pattison (ed.). *Clinical psychiatry and religion.* Boston: Little, Brown, 1969.

Weisner, W., & Riffel, A. Scrupulosity: Religion and obsessive compulsive behavior in children. *American Journal of Psychiatry,* 1960, *117,* 314-318.

Zilboorg, G. *Psychoanalysis and religion.* London: George Allen & Unwin, 1967.